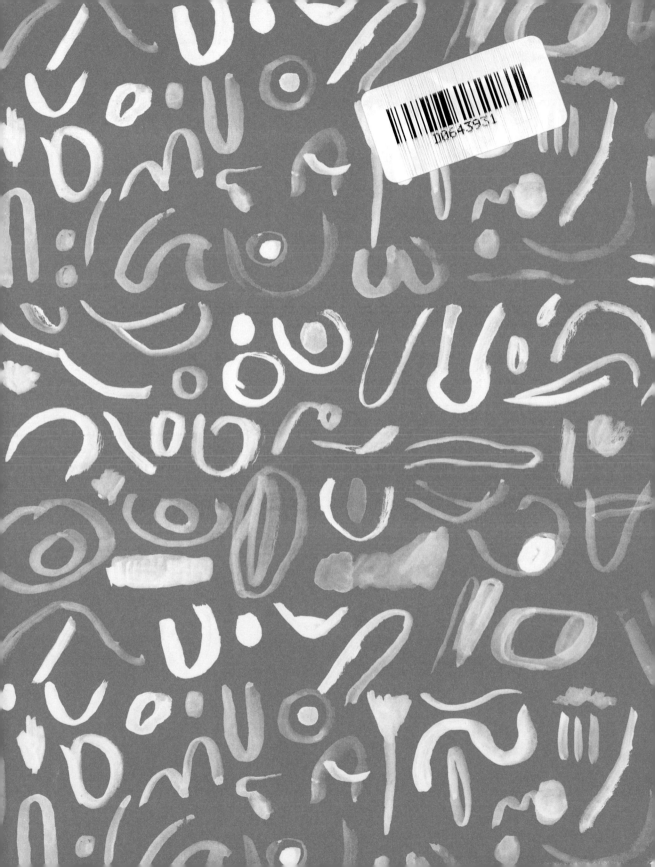

EVERY
BODY

An Honest and
Open Look at *SEX*
from Every Angle

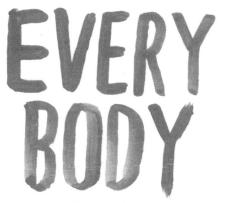

EVERY BODY

Julia Rothman
& Shaina Feinberg
& EVERYBODY

VORACIOUS

Little, Brown and Company

New York Boston London

Voracious / Little, Brown and Company
Hachette Book Group
1290 Avenue of the Americas, New York, NY 10104
littlebrown.com

First Edition: January 2021

Voracious is an imprint of Little, Brown and Company, a division of
Hachette Book Group, Inc. The Voracious name and logo are trademarks
of Hachette Book Group, Inc.

The publisher is not responsible for websites (or their content) that are not
owned by the publisher.

The Hachette Speakers Bureau provides a wide range of authors for
speaking events. To find out more, go to hachettespeakersbureau.com or
call (866) 376-6591.

All art and hand-lettering not separately credited by Julia Rothman

Book design by Jenny Volvovski

ISBN 978-0-316-42658-9
LCCN 2020936919

10 9 8 7 6 5 4 3 2 1

MOHN

Printed in Germany

For Mom:

thanks for letting me
ask you anything.
—Julia

For Chris:

thanks for loving my
heavy Jewish boobs.
—Shaina

CONTENTS

INTRODUCTION
How It Came Together *Julia Rothman* 9

STORY STATISTICS
An infographic representation of the
demographics of the contributors 12

STORIES
Learning About Sex 17

ESSAY
Jesus Dirt *Elna Baker* 23

STORIES
Masturbation 27

INTERVIEW: AS TOLD TO
Professional Masturbator *Betty Dodson* 33

STORIES
Body Acceptance 35

ESSAY
Dick *J. Colin Huerter* 41

STORIES
First Times 43

ESSAY
By the Sidewalk: A Memory *Fariha Róisín* 52

STORIES
Religion 55

ESSAY
Dating as a Muslim *Bilal Zafar* 62

STORIES
Race & Ethnicity 64

ESSAY
Lovemaking in the City of Dreams
Myles E. Johnson 67

STORIES
Mental Health 70

ESSAY
10 Things to Do When You're
Horny & Lonely *Fareeha Khan* 76

INTERVIEW: AS TOLD TO
Being Intersex *River Gallo* 80

STORIES
Sexual Identity, Orientation & Exploration 83

ESSAY
Just Me & My Assh*le *David Heatley* 94

INTERVIEW: AS TOLD TO
Living with HIV *Anonymous* 96

STORIES
STIs 99

ESSAY
What Does Jessica Rabbit Have That I Don't?
Rebekah Taussig 105

STORIES
Overcoming the Unexpected 109

INTERVIEW: AS TOLD TO
Sex Literacy *Erica Chidi Cohen* 117

STORIES
Whoops! What??? 121

STORIES
Dating & Hookups 129

ESSAY
Underwear Drop *Piera Gelardi* 133

STORIES
What I Like 135

ESSAY
Sex in Parks *Ren Khodzhayev* 143

STORIES
Location, Location, Location 147

STORIES
Infidelity 150

INTERVIEW: AS TOLD TO
What You Might See at a Sex Club
Anonymous 155

STORIES
Non-monogamy/Poly 159

STORIES
Group Sex & Sex Parties 162

ESSAY
A Taste of the Meat Rack! *Turdluv* 168

ESSAY
Bringing Up Daddy *Jude Dry* 172

STORIES
Fetish 175

INTERVIEW: AS TOLD TO
The Evolution of a Dominatrix
Mistress Velvet 182

STORIES
Sex Work 187

INTERVIEW: AS TOLD TO
Camming *Lauren Duck* 197

STORIES
Sex Toys 200

ESSAY
Answering the Question *Jiz Lee* 203

STORIES
Porn 207

ESSAY
The Fruit I Carry *Rachel Evans* 212

STORIES
Fertility, Pregnancy & Miscarriage 215

ESSAY
Things You Might Not Know About Miscarriage
Julia Wertz 222

INTERVIEW: AS TOLD TO
Teen Pregnancy *Anonymous* 226

STORIES
Abortions 230

ESSAY
Revolutionary Outlaw Lovers
Bianca I. Laureano, MA, CSES 234

INTERVIEW: AS TOLD TO
Life After a Sexual Assault *Karen Kornegay* 237

STORIES
Consent & Sexual Assault 241

INTERVIEW: AS TOLD TO
Forensic Sexologist *Eric Garrison* 250

ESSAY
No Sell-By Date *Gretta Keene, LCSW, CST* 253

STORIES
Aging 256

STORIES
COVID-19 259

CONCLUSION
Acorns *Shaina Feinberg* 267

ARTIST DIRECTORY 270

ACKNOWLEDGMENTS 271

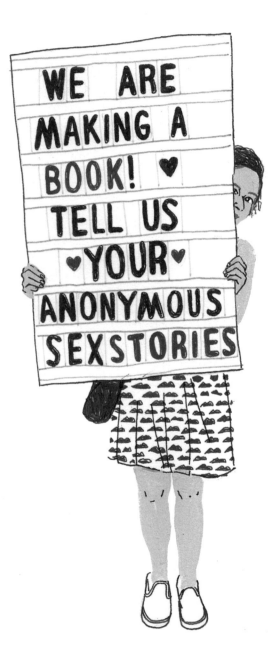

HOW IT CAME TOGETHER

by JULIA ROTHMAN

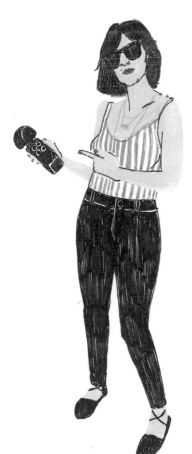

I read and listened to so many people's sex stories to make *Every Body,* and naturally those stories reminded me of my own experiences. As the collection came together I began to examine my entire sexual and romantic history, and I was full of questions: Why am I attracted to unavailable people? Why do I need sexual validation to feel good about myself? Should I experiment more? Am I weird for liking that? Had I given consent that time? What do I really want? Why am I alone?

I signed the deal for this book right after a breakup. I was single, I was missing my ex, and I was dating furiously—using a variety of apps. On first dates, I would mention that I was collecting sex stories to be published anonymously in a book. In response, many of the dates offered to tell me their stories. Some of them thought it would impress me to hear about their threesomes. One guy told me about his deformed penis. Another about slicing a girl's leg and drinking her blood before sex. I'd pull out my phone and start recording. After saying good night, I would rush home and transcribe.

I also collected stories for the book through a website, which I promoted via social media. On the website was a long drop-down menu of topics to choose from. Hundreds of stories came through pretty quickly. To guarantee a wide diversity of contributors, I requested personal data with each submission. Stories arrived from everywhere—across the country and other countries, too: Mexico, England, Australia, even Kazakhstan.

As the stories filtered in, I became overwhelmed and decided to bring on my friend Shaina to help me. Shaina is a filmmaker and is experienced at organizing wild projects. It was her idea that we go stand on the corner to solicit more stories. She thought we could interact with people in the street we wouldn't be able to reach through our networks. We made a sign that read TELL US YOUR ANONYMOUS SEX STORIES! I printed out consent forms; Shaina bought hand sanitizer.

Our first stop was Union Square, the hub of downtown Manhattan—where tons of people come in and out all day long. We sat on a bench with the sign propped against our legs. Shaina is fearless and would call out to people, "Can we talk to you about sex?" I was always quiet. A middle-aged man in a fedora sat down between us and admitted he was having an affair. He had been married for a very long time, but only since his affair had he finally understood love songs. A woman—it turned out she was a tourist from France—saw our sign and made a beeline for us. With trembling hands she told us how vaginismus prevents her from having sex with her new husband, and how she is seeking help from a hypnotist. Two women who had met in a halfway house told us about the sex work they'd done in the past. Shaina and I set goals. After we had spoken to twenty people in a location, we'd go home.

We collected stories all over New York City—the Fulton Mall, Coney Island, Washington Square Park. We flew to New Orleans and did the same thing in the French Quarter, where tons of people were walking. People would see our sign and run over to us, eager to share. At one point, a crowd had gathered. One guy compared having Viagra in his pocket to the feeling of having a loaded gun—which he knew all about, because he carries a loaded gun. Another woman described losing her virginity in a

Baptist church bathroom. And another told us how she explicitly educated her daughter (and all of her daughter's friends) about sex because her own mother had never mentioned it.

I was lucky enough to have a mom who talked to me about sex. When I was eleven years old, my mother sat me down and told me I could ask her anything about sex—*anything*. I am so grateful for her openness. My mom also gave me the book *Our Bodies, Ourselves*. In that book there are real stories interspersed with information. I loved reading those stories—people's secrets, their innermost feelings, their desires. I wanted to read more of those. I wanted a book made up exclusively of those stories.

So many of the stories that came in for this book were sad. Eventually—while soliciting stories—we had to ask specifically for "positive stories" because we had collected so many stories about abuse, loneliness, heartbreak, and fear. It was hard not to reach over and hug people when they teared up. Some people confided they had never told anyone what they were telling us. They said it felt good to share. Some people seemed disappointed when they were finished talking and we said goodbye.

I became obsessed with certain stories. I read them over and over—imagining the feelings the person was having, imagining having those feelings myself. I talked about the project in therapy. I talked about it with my mom. Why did I want to know people's intimate secrets? Why did I want to connect so intensely with everyone?

I thought about it. It's true I had no expertise, but I wanted to make this book because it didn't exist. Because not everyone had a mother like mine, who would sit them down and talk to them about sex. And because I wanted people to know they're not alone.

But I think the real reason might be more selfish: Ultimately I made this book so that *I* wouldn't feel alone. And it worked. I am forever grateful for everybody who shared their stories with me, with us, with you. Thank you.

LET US INTERVIEW YOU ABOUT SEX (ANONYMOUSLY) FOR A BOOK

STORY STATISTICS

For full transparency, here are the demographics we collected of all the people whose anonymous stories you will find in this book. The stories were collected through a submission form on a website and in-person conversations.

We tried our best to reach as much of the diverse population that would speak with us, but we will always strive to do better as we continue this project and others.

We can't guarantee the accuracy of these stories or demographics. These were all told to us, and we trust that the contributors were honest in their accounts. (We have changed all of the names in these accounts with the exception of those of the named contributors.)

GENDER

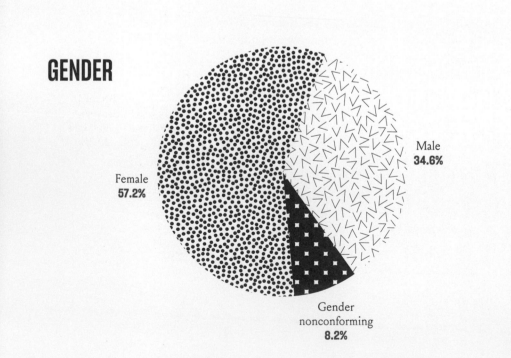

Female
57.2%

Male
34.6%

Gender
nonconforming
8.2%

AGE

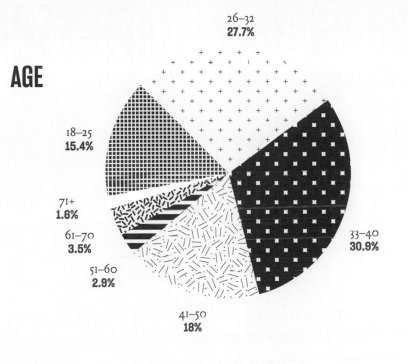

26–32
27.7%

18–25
15.4%

71+
1.6%

61–70
3.5%

51–60
2.9%

41–50
18%

33–40
30.9%

SEXUAL ORIENTATION

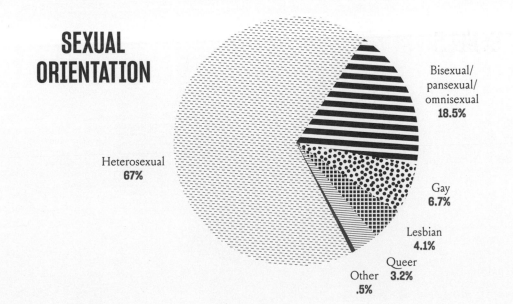

Heterosexual
67%

Bisexual/
pansexual/
omnisexual
18.5%

Gay
6.7%

Lesbian
4.1%

Queer **3.2%**

Other
.5%

ETHNICITY

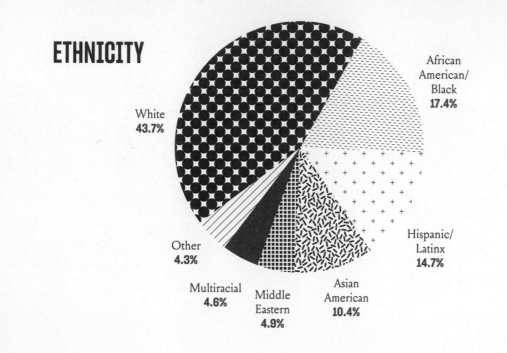

White
43.7%

African American/ Black
17.4%

Hispanic/ Latinx
14.7%

Asian American
10.4%

Middle Eastern
4.9%

Multiracial
4.6%

Other
4.3%

RELIGION

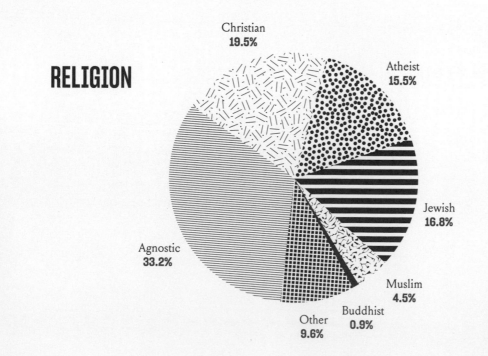

Christian
19.5%

Atheist
15.5%

Jewish
16.8%

Muslim
4.5%

Buddhist
0.9%

Other
9.6%

Agnostic
33.2%

LOCATION

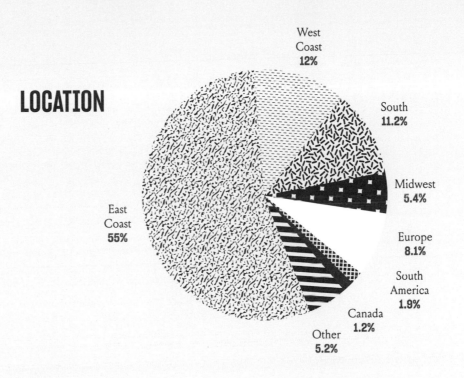

West
Coast
12%

South
11.2%

Midwest
5.4%

Europe
8.1%

South
America
1.9%

Canada
1.2%

Other
5.2%

East
Coast
55%

DISABILITY

We provided a fill-in-the-blank for the question: Do you have a disability?

0.5% of anonymous story contributors whose stories appear in this book wrote in that they do have a disability.

Heres a list of the things they wrote: Diabetes, Fibromyalgia, Lupus, HIV+, Ileostomy, Chronic Fatigue Syndrome, Parkinson's, Heart Defect, Bipolar disorder, PTSD.

LEARNING ABOUT SEX

SHAINA I first learned about sex from that book *Where Did I Come From?* I loved the pictures of the two chubby people having sex.

JULIA I had that book too! The people were so cute–remember they were in the bathtub together?

SHAINA Yes!

JULIA *How did you learn about sex?* was always the best question to ask people when we first approached them for stories on the street.

SHAINA Totally! It got the ball rolling!

JULIA I feel like it really took people back–they had to really think for a while.

In grade school, I think I was eight years old, we were learning about organisms in school. **And I was in the car with my dad and we had just driven into our garage and I guess I accidentally asked my dad, "What's orgasms?"** Then he was like, "Son, let me tell you…" and he spent half an hour with me in the garage talking about all this sex shit. My dad was a doctor. He was really point-blank and would answer in a very scientific way. And I was like, *whoa*—I didn't want to hear about that! I thought we were talking about *organisms*.

Sex ed came in high school. It was already way too late, though. We were already finger fucking by then. I remember hearing in sixth grade about a guy putting his hand down a girl's pants.

I learned about sex from this goth chick with huge tits in seventh grade. She told me everything I needed to know and showed me the way. We did it in a park. I lived in the suburbs then. My parents told me nothing about sex. My parents still think I'm a virgin—and I'm twenty-eight!

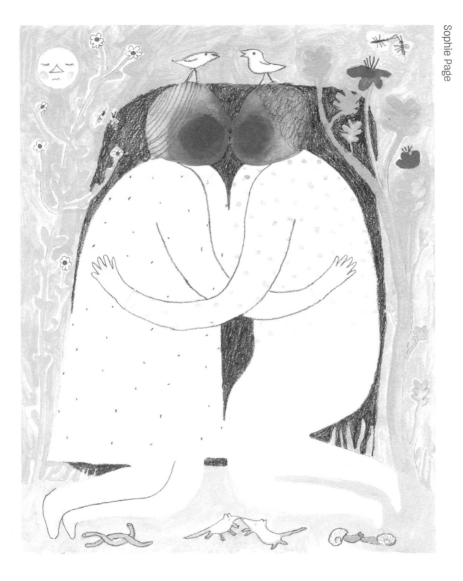

Sophie Page

My parents were highly sexual. My dad was not embarrassed to flaunt it in every aspect of his life. It's fair to say I first learned about sex from him—his behavior and mannerisms. We were a blue-collar family, lower middle class. The house was small. The rooms were next to each other. It wasn't a spacious house where my parents could tuck away and hide. My father had porn on VHS. Once I was twelve or thirteen, I became curious. I started snooping around my dad's room. It was almost instinctual. I knew there was something to find. I do specifically remember a first conversation where my dad asked me, "Are you having sex?" We were all gathered on their waterbed watching a flick and he posed the question. It was me, my mom, my sister. We were just hanging out. It was real casual. And I lied.

In Japan, there was no sex education. **No parents talk to their kids about sex. Ever.** They never say a word. It should all be secret. Yet there are porn movies and magazines everywhere. You can buy sexy cartoon magazines at 7 Eleven. When I was fifteen, my friends and I started watching porn. A lot of Japanese pornos use an octopus; they put it in a pussy. It's boiled and hardened. A lot of pornos use the tentacle legs. That was what I was watching as a kid.

I learned about sex from porno—old-school porno from the 1970s and '80s. **Hairy porno.** VHS porno.

My parents' idea of sex was very buttoned-up. We never had a conversation about sex. My dad told me when I was fourteen that an orgasm was like when you have to shit and you finally get to shit. And I was like, okay…? So I had a lot of shame about sex at first, but I've worked on being more open about it.

I had my first period when I was eleven years old. I didn't tell anybody. **My mom asked about it when she was doing laundry and found my bloody underpants.** I felt completely embarrassed about my periods for years. When my mom and sister were having "the talk" with me, I faked coughing the whole time because it made me feel so uncomfortable.

Nowadays I am okay with blood and tampons, but I feel more ashamed of the fact that I don't know anything about my natural cycle because I've been on the pill for half of my life.

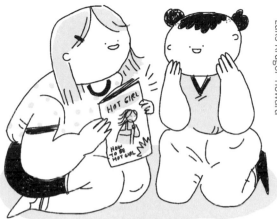

"Let's practice comparing our bodies to other people's bodies!"

I learned about sex by doing it. It felt good, so I did it. I'm of age. I'm not a kid. Nobody talked to women about sex back then. It was a responsibility, so we did it. It was the 1970s. I was in high school, everyone was doing it. So I did it. And I got pregnant. 1979. I had the baby. She's a grown-up now.

One of the things I tried to do with her growing up was to be more open about sex, explaining the parts and what the parts do and what feels good. I taught her and her friends. Like a community woman, like a Dr. Ruth. And then my daughter was like, "Ma, why did you do that?" But her friends were always like, "We love your mom, she talks real." I talked to them about masturbation. They were like, "What is *that*?" They cracked up. It was fun. We used to have Blockbuster [video] night—that's how long ago this was. I would tell her friends all about it. I was teaching about masturbating because as a woman you need to learn how to please yourself. Or else how are you going to teach your partner? That way you can guide him.

I grew up during the generation where sex wasn't talked about. So my friend Ava told me everything about sex — but it was all fucked up. She said if a boy touches your ass, you get pregnant. We were in grade school and we thought Ava knew every-thing. <u>Our classmate Dudley touched my butt and I thought I was pregnant.</u> I told my sister about it — I was really worried I was pregnant! But my sister told me the truth.

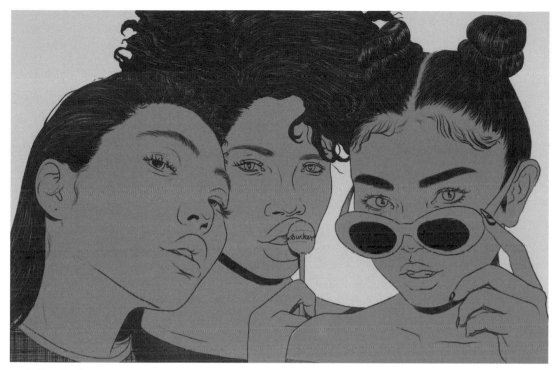

Rachelle Baker

Back in prehistoric times (the 1960s) when I attended a Catholic school, our sex education was talking to a priest for an hour. This was a big day for my fifth-grade class! All those mysterious rumors I had heard about the inconceivable and horrific activities my parents secretly participated in would be unveiled. Every day a kid was plucked out of our classroom and would return to their desk, quiet and slightly embarrassed. When they returned, I expected them to look different—maybe older and wiser?

My day finally came and I went to the rectory across from our school and sat in front of Father Schmidt, who was visibly uncomfortable and anxious. I honestly don't recall what he told me—it was basically biology and made no sense. The only thing I remember is ejaculation. I was alarmed to find out that something other than urine came out of my penis. I persisted in asking him questions about it long after he wanted to move on to another topic. His irritability was showing. "What is this stuff—sperm? Does it hurt? What's it look like?

Can you stop it if you want? How much comes out?" I must have asked that last one three times. Finally, Father Schmidt said, "It's white, and it's about a tablespoon." I silently winced in horror. Ten minutes later I returned to the class. **My sex education was over and I felt more confused than before.**

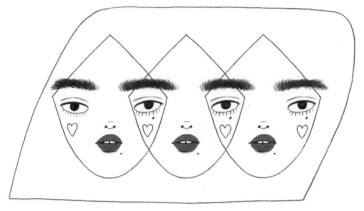

Manjit Thapp

I got the best lesson from my parents about sex. **They said the one thing we want you to know about sex is you've done nothing if your partner isn't happy.** That was before anything. Before I learned about the birds and the bees. Just understanding that this is a very intimate thing that happens between two people. And both people have to be engaged and enjoying it. I think that has a lot to do with how picky I am. I won't just take any woman. She has to be like a dope in so many ways and a great counterpoint to who I am. And really know herself. So much of the sex you see on TV is meaningless and between two people who barely know each other.

I went to a private international school in Ethiopia. We were in fifth grade. Class was canceled for a week. **And in that time we had other classes devoted to sex and puberty and our bodies.** We weren't learning about pleasure or masturbation. It was more of the physical aspects: these are the types of sex, this is what your body is doing. I think it helped me compare to what I hear Americans say about sex ed. I didn't have any of the stigma or shame around having sex. I'm very open about talking about sex.

When I was sixteen, I told my mom I was ready for birth control—and, therefore, sex. She kept her cool but quickly threw away my idea. **No matter how many times I talked to her, she never took me to a gyno.** Years later, when I was twenty, I got pregnant. Although I love my now-four-year-old son with all my heart, I really tried to reach my mom for help when I was a teenager, when I didn't have a single clue about sex at all. It would be nice to change parents' minds when it comes to *preserve a daughter from sex* (my mom's words). Sex is natural, sex can be safe, and it's a part of everyone's life.

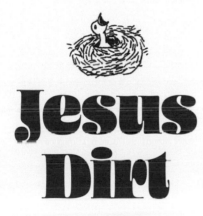

Jesus
Dirt

by ELNA BAKER

I had recently seen the documentary *The Devil's Playground,* which is about Amish kids and how at sixteen they have a *Rumspringa* where they go out into the world and do anything they want to with no religious consequences—I decided that I would take a one-year break from being Mormon (this, by the way, is totally not allowed). But I decided the only way to know if it was true was to leave and then come back to it.

My plan was to go wild. I had an imaginary list of men I would sleep with. But the second I was free to do whatever I wanted, I couldn't.

It was like there was an invisible electric fence around me. The closer I got, the more paralyzed I became. Especially when it came to sex. In Mormonism you're taught that sexual sin before marriage is the second most serious sin next to murder. You're told that if you engage in it you won't be allowed to be with your family in the afterlife. I'd had some sexual experiences before, but never anything more than groping—and that one time my neighbor kissed the outside of the crotch of my pajama pants and I'd had an orgasm.

I'd become a regular at this tiny bar/dance club called the Beatrice. During the first few months of my break I'd go there almost every other night, meet a guy, and we'd go back to his place and make out. I'd want to do more. He'd want me to do more. I'd stare at the bulge in his pants and think about touching it. But that just seemed rude. Inappropriate. So I wouldn't do anything. It was a mixture of the religious stuff—*this is murder, I'll lose my family*—and plain old insecurity: I was scared of being bad at it. I was twenty-seven, an age by which people expect you to be sexually experienced. No one would ever guess I was doing things for the first time. Which meant that if I was bad at sex, or blow jobs, or hand jobs, they'd just think I sucked. They wouldn't know it was my first time. And this fear of being inexperienced kept me from *getting* experience. I'd inch closer and closer to the dick, but chicken out and leave abruptly.

After months of doing this, I confided in my friend Andy.

"I have a close friend who left Orthodox Judaism in his mid-twenties," Andy told me. "He went through a lot of the same things. I'm going to introduce you. I bet he'd be a helpful person to talk to about this."

I met David at a small Italian restaurant in the West Village, one where you had to walk downstairs to get in. It was dimly lit with candles and had the kind of ambience that just feels sexy. He was cute. I'd googled him beforehand, but he was hotter in person. He had an energy about him—like he was aware that he was in charge. During my Google search I'd read some articles he'd written. He was a very accomplished writer, which made him seem older and cooler than me. But right when I sat down I felt comfortable. We talked for two hours. He told me about his decision to leave. And asked me questions about mine. I told him about my concern that my family would find out and it'd be heartbreaking for them. And about my anxieties and the fear of making a choice I couldn't take back, which at this point had become paralyzing.

"I felt the same way when I left," he said. "How long have you been out?"

"About five months," I said. Not clarifying I was technically not out at all.

"You're exactly where you're supposed to be. It's going to take a lot longer than you think to get used to everything. Don't feel the need to rush it. Be patient with yourself."

"Yes, but I have only a year."

"What do you mean?"

I leaned in. As the candle flickered in his brown eyes, I went into detail about my decision to take a *Rumspringa* and my plan to potentially return to Mormonism at the end of the year. He found this amusing.

"So you're on a break."

"Exactly."

"And what have you done so far?"

"What do you mean?"

"Have you been drinking?"

"No."

"What about drugs? Any drugs?"

"No."

"What about sex? Have you had sex yet?"

I looked into his eyes not wanting to answer. "Honestly? I have no idea what to do with a penis."

He stared back at me, unflinchingly. And then, looking directly into my eyes, he said, "Do you want me to show you?" (He said this like it was some form of community service all formerly religious people had to do.)

I bit my lip. This was maybe the sexiest thing that had ever happened to me.

"Yes," I said.

Within ten minutes we'd settled up, hailed a cab, and were back in my apartment. We sat nervously on the couch, with the lights on, staring straight ahead.

"You've *seen* a penis before, right?" he asked me.

"Yes," I said, with a little too much bravado to sound believable. It was true. Sort of. I'd changed diapers before. So, baby dicks. I'd seen baby dicks.

Now here I was, about to see the real thing—the adult version. I tried to mentally prepare myself so I didn't make the wrong face. Not that I knew what the right face was. David turned and looked at me, as if to say, *Are you ready?* I nodded my head yes. He unzipped his pants and slid them down a little. Then he reached into his underwear and took out his dick. I looked at it with wide-eyed wonder.

"It's so big," I accidentally blurted out. (And it was. Compared with, say, a baby's dick.)

"Wow," he said. "You're already good at this."

What followed was partly erotic, partly instructional. First, David gave me a guided tour of his dick. "This part here is called the head," he said. He gestured to each section as he spoke: "This is called the shaft. These are the balls."

"And you're not supposed to touch those," I said. I was basing this information on *America's Funniest Home Videos.* When men got kicked in the balls they always fell over. So it seemed like balls were off-limits.

"No, you can touch the balls." He took my hand and placed it on his balls.

"They're so soft," I said. "Like a baby bird."

We both cringed.

I lifted my hand. It hovered over his penis for a second. I wanted to touch it. But I was too afraid.

"It's okay," he said. "You can touch it."

I touched it lightly with one finger, the way you

might wipe ketchup off someone's face if you didn't know them very well: cautious but kind.

"Here," he said, taking my hand and wrapping it around the base of his penis. "You can be a lot more firm with it." He put his hand around mine to show me the amount of pressure. Then he took his hand away. I held on a little tighter.

"Not that firm," he corrected me. And I wanted to die.

"If you move your hand up and down the penis, it feels really good," he explained. "But you need moisture."

David spit into his hand—like a *ton* of spit—and rubbed it onto his penis. I had to actively control the face I wanted to make: *What? You just spit on your penis!*

From here he took my hand in his and showed me the speed and pressure I should use when I stroked his dick. After a minute he took his hand away so I could do it on my own, and then every thirty seconds he'd put it back to help me stay on rhythm. It was a bit like learning to drive—if you were using only the stick shift.

"Yeah. That's it," he said, encouraging me. "And now go a little faster." My hand bobbed up and down in the narrow space between us. It occurred to me how strange it was that this was happening. We hadn't even kissed yet. So I leaned in toward him, and he kissed me. We kissed for a little bit. Our tongues pressed together in synch with the bobbing of my hand. I pulled back a little and looked into his big brown eyes. He looked back into mine.

"Do you ever get over the guilt?" I asked. The second I asked that, I knew it was the wrong thing to say. His expression can best be described by that record-scratching-to-a-halt sound effect.

His penis, which had felt strong and firm against my hand, suddenly turned into a limp noodle. I struggled to get a grip on it. I now know that this is called *losing an erection,* but at the time I had no idea what was going on.

"What's happening?" I said, in a panic. "Did I hurt you? Are you okay?"

"No," he tried to reassure me. "It's not you." We both moved around awkwardly. He took my hand off his penis and set it back in my lap with a little pat, as if to say, *You stay there.*

Then he tucked his penis back into his underwear. "I...I don't think we should do this," he said.

"No!" I said. "I'm totally fine—I want to do this. I'm sorry. I shouldn't have said that." I tried to pull him back toward me, but he blocked my advances.

"It's not your fault. I thought you were further along than you are. I'm sorry. I had a great night. And I don't mean to make you feel embarrassed." He was trying to be nice, but it was undermined by the fact that he was rushing to collect his things and heading to the door like there was a fire. He kissed me goodbye, but it was a polite kiss—one you'd give your aunt. And then he left. No *What's your number?* No *Hey, I'd like to see you again.*

The second David was gone, I could feel the Mormon guilt surging up from the back of my head like a migraine about to set in. *No.* I tried to will it back down. *Just stop thinking. Don't think.*

I rushed into the bathroom and downed two sleeping pills. As I drifted off to sleep, it all felt a little like a dream. And not a good one. *What's wrong with me?*

I woke up the next morning paralyzed with fear. And this is when the brainwashing really went into full effect. I'd broken the first major rule. This was different from letting someone lightly graze your boob over the bra; this was a serious sexual sin. By touching a penis, I had tarnished my very soul and would never be the same person again. I'd been trained for nearly two decades to associate premarital sex with murder, and this belief was embedded deep within my subconscious.

I tried to stop the thoughts from coming. I even gave myself a little pep talk: *It's okay... you're okay...it's all going to be okay. So you touched a penis. The world didn't end. No one died. It's not that big a deal.*

It helped. A little. But as I climbed down the ladder of my loft bed, with each progressive step I felt like I was getting closer to the reality of what I'd done. Last night was real. I couldn't take it back. I could never undo it. The second my feet hit the floor, all my religious guilt came flooding in and I collapsed to the ground in tears. It was the kind of display of grief that is usually reserved for the death of a loved one. *What have I done?*

It's hard to explain this to people who weren't raised with the same dogmatic beliefs, because to them it all seems so silly. What had I done? I'd touched a penis. *No big deal,* right? But in my mind I had done something truly horrible. It was as if I'd committed a crime. I was bad. I was evil. I was an impure woman. And God was deeply disappointed in me. I knew better. And yet I'd fallen for Satan and the temptations of my flesh. And in doing so I'd also defiled the body of another person, and I could never take that back.

But it wasn't just guilt and remorse—it was fear. I was breathing heavily, panting through the tears. It was as if I'd ventured into the forest alone at night and a monster was chasing me. It was the inexplicable feeling that I'd opened myself up to danger or harm. Because that's what happens to the slutty girls, isn't it? It's the images we grow up with, the ones we see over and over again that lay the foundations for our beliefs. It wasn't just Mormonism. In the world at large, female sexuality is linked to violence. Often this violence comes to women who are just walking home at night. It's less a result of exercising their sexuality than merely existing. But the message we get as young girls is that the women who want it get what they have coming. I'd been taught that if I was chaste and pure, I'd be watched over by God—protected from this violence. This of course is an illusion, but I'd bought into it. And now this protective veil was gone. Anything could happen to me now.

Lying in this pathetic puddle on the ground, crying, I had an idea. It wasn't even a Mormon belief, it was just a crazy thought my own head invented. When I was seventeen, we'd gone on a family trip to Jerusalem and visited the Garden of Gethsemane. This was the exact spot where the atonement of Christ took place. Here Jesus had bled for the sins of all mankind. And through this loving act of self-sacrifice, we can be forgiven for any sins so long as we repent of them. While I was there, I had collected a ziplock bag of dirt from the garden. When I got back home, I bought a pale-green glass vase and filled it with this dirt. I kept it in the display cabinet in my living room to remind me of the sacrifice Jesus had made for me.

And so, as if it were the most normal thing in the world—routine, as though a doctor had prescribed it as a cure—I walked over to the cabinet and took down the vase of dirt. I poured a handful of the Jesus dirt into my penis-touching hand and said a prayer: *Dear Heavenly Father, through the blood of Christ that is in this dirt forgive me for touching David's penis. I would like to repent for this sin. I promise I will never do it again. I say these things in the name of Jesus Christ. Amen.*

I held both my hands out, then rubbed them together like I was washing my hands with dirt. Then I stood over the garbage can and symbolically dropped the dirt in. It was my sacrifice. Because I'd done something so bad, I had to give some of my dirt away in order to be forgiven. And the craziest part about it was...*it worked.* This invented-on-the-spot ritual gave me the tiniest bit of relief. I could breathe. I had hope again. There was forgiveness for these sins.

But here's the problem with sexual curiosity: it's like a drumbeat building inside you, getting faster and faster. And wherever you left off last, you can't stop until you get back there—and go a little bit further. So where once there was Jesus dirt, two weeks later there was another dick in my hand.

MASTURBATION

JULIA Reading stories about masturbation–it's amazing how resourceful people are! So many people used hairbrushes!

SHAINA Yeah! And toothbrushes. And stuffed animals. And bedposts!

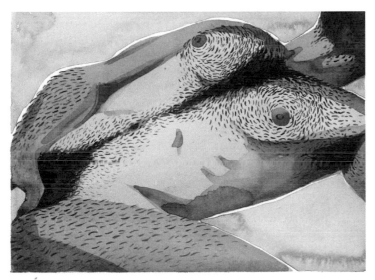

October Joe

When I was in camp, I learned how to masturbate. I asked someone, **"Do you just lick your hand and touch it?"** That didn't work. The only thing I had to use was toothpaste. As a twelve-year-old, you don't know much yet. So I put toothpaste on my dick and started rubbing, and it felt really good. Then I was like, "Shit! It stings—it stings!" That was a good lesson.

I used to go to the Fort Greene farmers market in Brooklyn on Saturdays, and one time this guy started to talk to me; he was a farmer and had a stand there. We were talking for two hours. About everything. **I just couldn't leave his three-foot radius.** He had to take care of his customers, but he didn't even look at them—he just kept talking to me. I've never felt so connected to a stranger before. I could have married him right there and then.

Before we said goodbye, I bought some vegetables from him. He wanted to give them to me for free, but I insisted. When I got home, glowing from this experience, I looked at this cucumber he grew upstate, grabbed it—it felt right—and had sex with the cucumber at 3 p.m., the sun shining right at me on the bed.

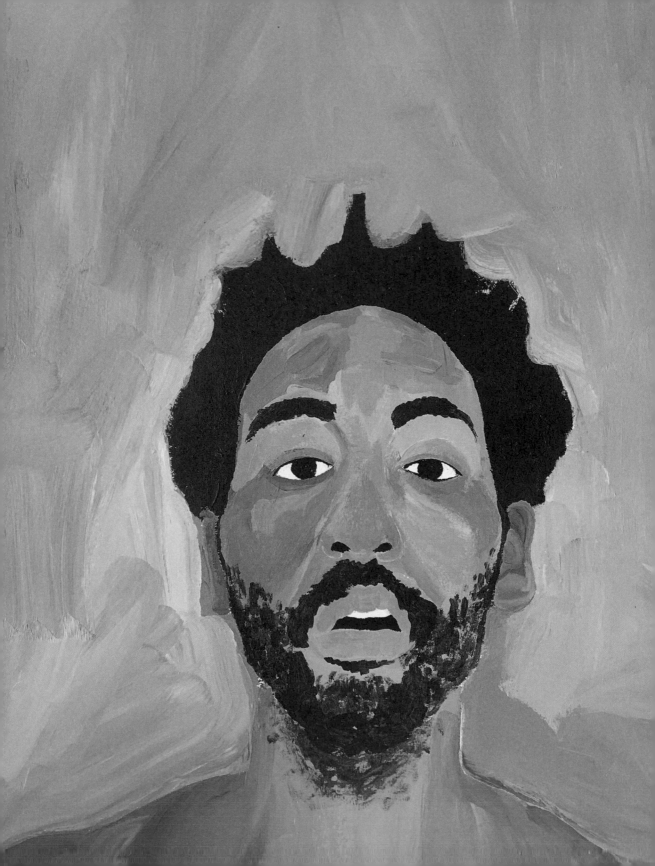

When I was about three or four, I was in a Montessori preschool at a church. We had nap time, playground time, crafts, and so on. It was all the usual stuff, except that I was one horny little kid. I remember showing my vagina to my two best friends in the little house on the playground. They showed me their penises. **I'm not sure if I touched myself at all, but I know I orgasmed in preschool.**

We had nap time on these rough cots in the basement of the church. They gave us little blankets. I lay facedown on the cot and did what I often did at home: I put both my hands on my vagina and kind of squirmed around until it happened. The problem was that the cot rubbed my little nose raw as I masturbated—it was bleeding! I do not totally know how the adults handled this, or if they figured out how it happened. I do know my mother was aware of what a sexual kid I was.

She once caught me lazing around in my bed at probably age five or six with some of her lotions lying around. I was putting them on my vagina because I liked how they felt. She just looked angry, took the lotions back, and said nothing. Sometimes, as an adult, I kind of wonder what else she knew.

She used to sit on the edge of my bed, dozing because I was afraid to fall asleep in the dark without her. Occasionally when she was there at her perch, I masturbated facedown. I think it was probably pretty imperceptible. I still masturbate in a version of this position, and I know it's pretty nonobvious. But I wonder if she knew, why didn't she say anything? Was she willfully ignoring it?

When I got older, my childhood best friend joined in on the fun. We met in kindergarten and started having sleepovers. We used to make "soup." We used all the kitchen implements from our respective play-food sets to fake-cut our vaginas,

pretending to scoop the cut pieces into the soup. We'd fake-cut each other's vaginas too.

When we got to high school, she used to tease me about the soup in public. We weren't really friends anymore, just friendly. No one would have known what she was talking about, but I was so embarrassed by it. Why was she so much more comfortable than me with what we did as kids? Maybe it was because she had a boyfriend and I did not. I had a lot of body-image issues at that age, too.

I still wonder about the normalcy of my masturbation habits and how they came to be. I know now that plenty of girls start masturbating young, but I was *very* young. I also loved it! I did it all the time. In my preteen years, I had a strong desire to shove penis-shaped objects inside me before I even knew much about penises. I also started feeling attracted to older boys and men. I started fantasizing about being dominated. I have no idea how or why this started.

As a preteen, most other girls wanted these sweet romances, like in the movies. I just craved rough sex. I never dreamed of getting married or having children. I still don't. I lie to men about this all the time. My sexuality has just always felt different from other straight women's. So have my relationship goals. It has led to a lot of confusion and unhappiness.

This all just makes me miss how I used to masturbate as a young child. It was really innocent then. It didn't have to mean anything. It just sprung up out of nowhere. It was unattached to relationships or other people's judgment. It was my private activity. It wasn't practice for later, or a placeholder for sex. Now my orgasms feel expected by men, even when I don't have them. Someone is waiting for them, and my escape—my lack of control—is gone.

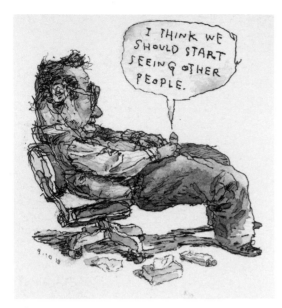

John Cuneo

Let's go way back to my very first masturbation. I was fifteen years old, and living with my parents in a small town on the East Coast. Mom's second-generation Roman Catholic Polish; Dad's conservative Chinese/ Malaysian.

I snuck into the living room to watch HBO while my parents slept. At this time it was a common practice for me to scan the TV guide (yes, that's how long ago this was!) for anything that could be sex-related. Coincidentally, that's how I got into *Sex and the City,* because the guide could fit only the words *Sex and.* But that was good enough for me!

Tonight, fifteen-year-old me was there to watch *G-String Divas.* This magical show highlighted four strippers working at a club. It showed them onstage and backstage, laughing, joking, getting dressed, dancing. It was femme friendship—helping, bonding. It was the sex-positive community of my dreams.

And then there was Hope. Hope had a boyfriend…and a girlfriend. There were clips of Hope talking to the camera, real world–style. Here she is kissing her boyfriend, and here kissing her girlfriend. My mind was blown. This was all possible?

I learned more useful information about sex and relationships in the first fifteen minutes of that show than I had learned in fifteen years of sex ed. Now, I'm sure the primary goal for the producers of *G-String Divas* was to help some small-town girl, struggling with her sexuality, find acceptance and a sex-positive femme community. But some other aspects of the show also caught my eye.

The stripping. Of course, the stripping. Here were these now–role models to me who were also fine as hell. And I'm sure there were audience members and men that they were dancing for, but in my view they were dancing just for me.

When the show ended, I felt like I had been through something. An experience. **And I was suddenly overwhelmed with a sensation that I knew I needed to do something about.** So I went down to my teenage room in the basement. I pushed aside my beaded curtains and put my Destiny's Child CD into my boom box. And I started to search.

I don't know how my young mind knew what I was looking for. I didn't really have any sexual experience besides making out, but heteronormative is pervasive. I pulled out any object that I thought might work, dismissing each one, until I found it. *It* was a round hairbrush, the kind with bristles all around, and a round, pink, plastic handle. "That'll do," I thought to myself.

I lay down on the dolphin comforter on my twin bed, staring at my Hanson posters, and I had to pause. The rush had worn off in the time it took me to find an object. But as soon as I started thinking about Hope—her girlfriend, the dancing—it all came rushing back. I grabbed that hairbrush by the bristles and just started shoving.

I'm not saying I had my first orgasm that night, but some time later, when the wave had passed, I returned to my body and slowly stopped moving. I took the hairbrush out, lay back flat on my bed, and thought, *What...the hell...was that?*

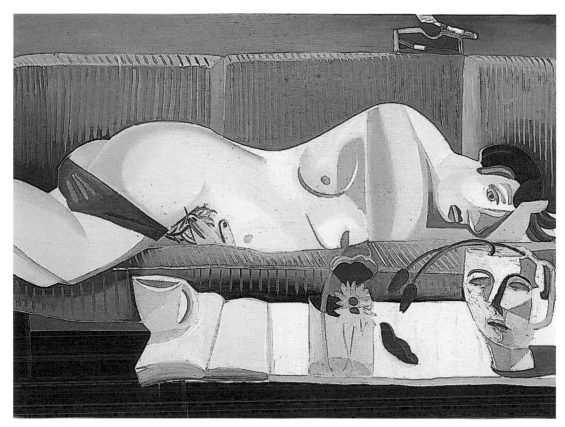

Danielle Orchard

I masturbate to porn a lot. It started when I was younger, maybe eight or nine. I heard about it somewhere—I'm not sure where—and looked up how girls masturbated, because I'd never been taught it in school. I remember thinking it kind of hurt to orgasm but was also nice. I masturbated with an electric toothbrush. I'd also heard about porn and erotica, so I tried looking them up. I discovered what I was "into" and got off by watching that.

Fast forward to five or six years later, when I still masturbated at least weekly, using the flat end of the head of the brush like I always had. But I never really could orgasm alone as well as I could when I was watching porn. So one day, home alone, I decided to just focus on where it felt good and how it felt rather than focusing on what outward things turned me on—like porn. It made me orgasm much better than any porn or erotica had.

Personal note: I am Christian and I have never thought that my love for God is defined by how much I choose to pleasure myself sexually. I feel they are completely different things, like how much you like ice cream versus how much you like cake. God loves me eternally and wants me to love myself too, and this is a form of self-love.

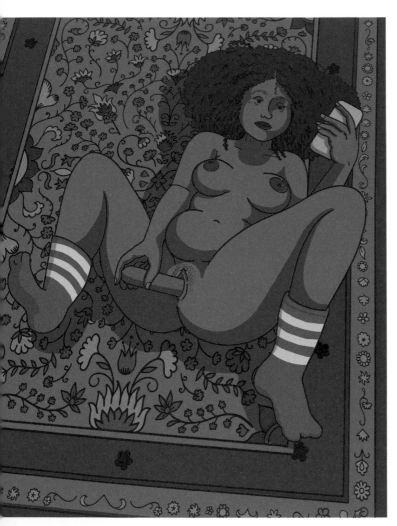

Siobhan Gallagher

I usually masturbate every day. I'll stop masturbating for five days in a row sometimes so I can get my drive really going.

I use olive oil to masturbate. It has a good consistency. It's not too light. It's not too heavy, but heavy enough. It's easy to clean up. It's natural. **And who's going to question why you have olive oil in the house?**

When I masturbate, the quicker I can get it done, the better. I think of it as a temperature drop needing to happen in my body. I need some stimulation—a porn video. The most important thing is the sound. I like watching too, voyeuristically, but the sound is key. It's important that the video feels real. I want to hear what they are saying and the environment. If there's no sound in the video, it's totally disconnected—it doesn't work. I might as well not watch anything.

When I was a kid, I was really good at climbing. I used to climb the poles on the playground really easily, a thousand times. One time I realized it started to give me pleasure. **When I came up the pole, I felt really good in an explosive way.**

I told my mom about my discovery and she told me that it was great, just not to do it when people were around.

Some time after, I realized these were orgasms, and that it was really easy for me to touch my body and "get there."

PROFESSIONAL MASTURBATOR

BETTY DODSON

I'm Betty Dodson, and I'm a professional masturbator—that is, I teach groups how to masturbate. How I got to teaching masturbation was a progression. I can't give you a time when all of a sudden I was an expert; it was always in my life.

I always talked about sex in school, and as a young adult I was always interested in it. As an artist, I was always drawing the nude form. And sex—It's such a good feeling. But masturbation—now *that* is great! It's free. You can do it alone or with friends. It's the perfect kind of sex.

And I love teaching groups how to masturbate. I love gathering a group of people and teaching them what I know. I love masturbating with them. The orgasm you have in those groups—it's heavenly. Because the energy in the room is incredible. Listen, I'm almost ninety and I still masturbate, but I'm done with having sex in a couple—once you teach masturbation to a group of people and masturbate with them, having sex in a couple is boring.

When I was a kid of about four or five, I was in the back seat of the car with my family—three brothers and me and my mom. I waited until my brothers had dozed off, then I stuck my fingers down my pants and started rubbing myself and it felt great and I had an orgasm. And then I noticed that my mom could see me in the rearview mirror. It probably wasn't my first orgasm, but it was certainly my first *observed* orgasm. But the interesting thing is that my mom didn't stop me. Back then all mothers were stopping kids from playing with themselves—well, I'm sure they still are, actually. But my mom didn't stop me. When I asked her about it later, she said, *Well, you were having so much fun and you weren't hurting anyone—and it was a long drive!* That was a beautiful answer. That's what I'm trying to teach other people about masturbation—you're not hurting anyone, and it's fun!

Here's something to remember when it comes to masturbation: penetration plus vibration. It's easy to remember because it rhymes. And when it comes to vibration, I am particularly fond of the Hitachi Magic Wand. It does the trick. If you want to get started somewhere, go to a sex shop. They have all kinds of things and the staff is usually informed.

When folks want to know my turn-ons, I say my biggest turn-on is *me*. I'm crazy about myself, but I wasn't always—I was insecure. As I got older and did more and accomplished more, however, I got more confident. A good tip for getting into yourself is don't compare yourself to anyone else. Ever. I truly believe in that. It works.

My personal philosophy is this: I think that giving yourself an orgasm is the heart of female liberation. Here's why: it's about knowing yourself, not depending on anyone else (independence!), and being in touch with your physical self. You have access to pleasure whenever you want it! Remember that! You can have an orgasm whenever you want to! That is freedom. Sexual freedom. But a lot of people are repressed—you can thank religion for that. In my workshops we spend a lot of time telling our stories first, and they are so similar. Repression has similarities.

Most of us had sex games as kids, and that is completely natural: *I'll show you mine if you show me yours.* But it's so surprising how conservative people are, how fearful, and how programmed they are. We're always discouraging kids about exploring their bodies. Why? Society has a lot of growing up to do. And I think it will happen. I think it's happening now—slowly, very slowly, but little by little it is happening. And we will be more open-minded.

Right now the culture is so focused on monogamy. I don't believe in monogamy. I never wanted to have sex with just one person. It's like eating the same food all the time. Variety is the spice of life—it's an old saying, but true. I was married for about five years in my late twenties. Then my marriage ended and I was outwardly sad, but inside I was happy—it was freedom! I belonged to the world!

I get asked all the time how I "identify": *How do you identify?* Well, there are all of these words now, but when I was younger we didn't have these terms. And to me it's irrelevant what your sexual preference is when you're talking about masturbation. Because you're having sex with yourself! I'm a solo sexual, that's what I am. And when I'm not being a solo sexual, I'm being a social sexual. It's not about hetero- or homosexual for me; it's either solo or social. People would be less judgmental if they thought that way. Why don't we all just be who we are!

People could really benefit from being less judgmental in general—about themselves and everyone else. Like with bodies—once you start having sex in a group, you see a lot of bodies and they're all just fine. You get accepting of all kinds of bodies once you see a lot of them naked. Try it!

BODY ACCEPTANCE

SHAINA Body acceptance is something that I still struggle with at times.

JULIA I still struggle with it too. I go through periods of caring about my weight obsessively, then sometimes not at all. I thought I would grow up and not care, but it creeps back sometimes. It's been helpful that as a society we are talking about it more.

When I was nineteen, I started to go bald. That was the same time I started to grow a lot of body hair. This felt like a crisis, that I was going bald that young—that girls wouldn't like me. And the body hair started growing on my back and on my butt—a lot of it. I was very embarrassed, but I didn't know what I could do about it. I couldn't have shaving my butt become part of my daily grooming routine. I was always afraid to let anyone see me from behind when I was naked because of my butt hair. But eventually I got over it and learned to live with it. I didn't really have another choice.

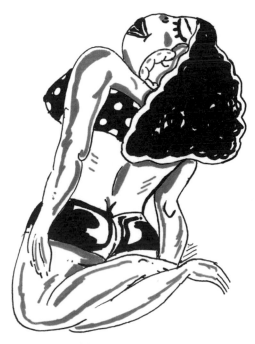

Do your labia minora hang low, do they wobble to and fro? **I have always been self-conscious of my vagina because my vaginal lips are big and sag a lot.** Also, the color is a lot darker. It's almost like extra elbow skin. They've been like that since I can remember. When I was younger, my high-school friend saw my vagina when we were changing or peeing or something, and she asked me if I had a penis. That was really traumatizing. I thought something was wrong with me down there. I still kind of do. I always wonder if guys pause when they see my long lips. Nobody has ever said anything. Eventually I asked my gyno and he said it was normal, but I'm still worried about it.

Branche Coverdale

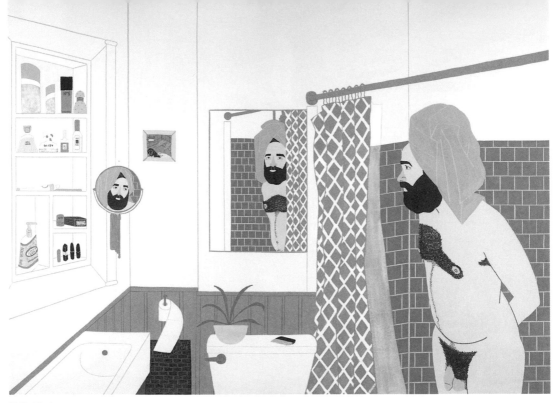

Kelly Bjork

I have inverted nipples. For as long as I can remember, every single time I went to a doctor they were like, *"How long have you had inverted nipples?!"* I guess it can be a symptom of breast cancer.

I would always say, "I've always had them."

And then they'd be like, "Oh, okay—well, you probably won't be able to nurse."

Doctors have been saying that to me since I was practically a kid—like way before I was ever gonna be nursing anyone. It gave me a complex. **I thought there was something wrong with my boobs. I honestly felt like a monster.** I would worry—as a teenager—about having to go skinny-dipping or something like that, and people seeing my inverted nipples. When I had sex or was changing in front of people, I would always cover them up. This went on for years and years and years.

Then, the night I got engaged, my fiancé was like, "I know you have a thing about your nipples, so just show me now so we can get over it." Like, that's how much of a complex I had! I had gotten engaged without even showing him my nipples. So I showed him my nipples, and it was no big deal—he thought they were cool. He also told me he had seen inverted nipples before, and they were great. (He's a boob man, so he just likes boobs.)

Anyway, after that I felt better about my boobs. And then when I got pregnant, all the doctors I went to were like, "You may not be able to nurse," and I was like, "Okay." Then I had my kid—and he sucked the nipples right out! I nursed him until he was two and a half years old, and I made so much milk I even donated some to people who needed it. So, the doctors were wrong after all: ain't nothing wrong with an inverted nipple.

I went on a date with a guy a few months ago, and I told him I'd recently had surgery. His response was, "Did you get an extra nipple removed?" It really bothered me and was not a good way to start a date.

"No," I laughed.

The surgery was not for that, but the truth is I *have* had extra nipples: **I was born with four nipples.** They are both underneath my boobs. They don't look like nipples. One was bigger than the other and stuck out more. Growing up, I wanted to wear bikinis because I was a skinny girl, but I also felt really self-conscious. Any time I was in a bra and a friend saw, they would ask me what it was. I would just say it was nothing or try to cover it up. I would wear tankinis to the beach.

At some point, maybe when I was ten, my mom took me to a dermatologist to ask if I could get them removed. They "burned them off" but in actuality it made them worse, because they were burned but still there. Then in high school, I really wanted the bigger one removed. The doctors supposedly cut it out, but now I have a scar and three stitches, and it still clearly looks to me like a nipple underneath.

The fourth one is still there—I just tell people it's a birthmark. I've become much more comfortable with it over the years, and I wear bikinis now. Sometimes if I feel close to people, I tell them what it is. For example, I wound up telling that guy—our date got better—and he was very surprised; he said he never would have known that's what that was.

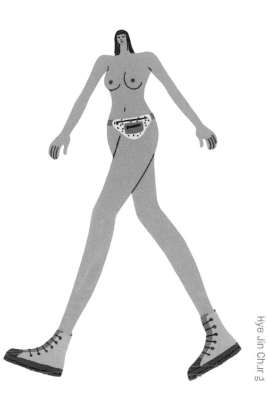

Hye Jin Chung

The first time I took my clothes off for someone, I worried about my breast symmetry, pubic-hair grooming, and most of all the stretch marks that looked to me like scarred-over claw marks running ribbons up my sides. **I had no reason to worry, because I was absolutely adored from head to toe.** Without me mentioning these blemishes, the person I love pointed them out as beautiful shimmering stripes. He did not have the term *stretch marks* in his mind and just saw them as they were. I have never seen myself the same way since.

P.S. That was almost twenty years ago. I married that person, who still challenges every unkind thing I try to think about myself with devout love and lust.

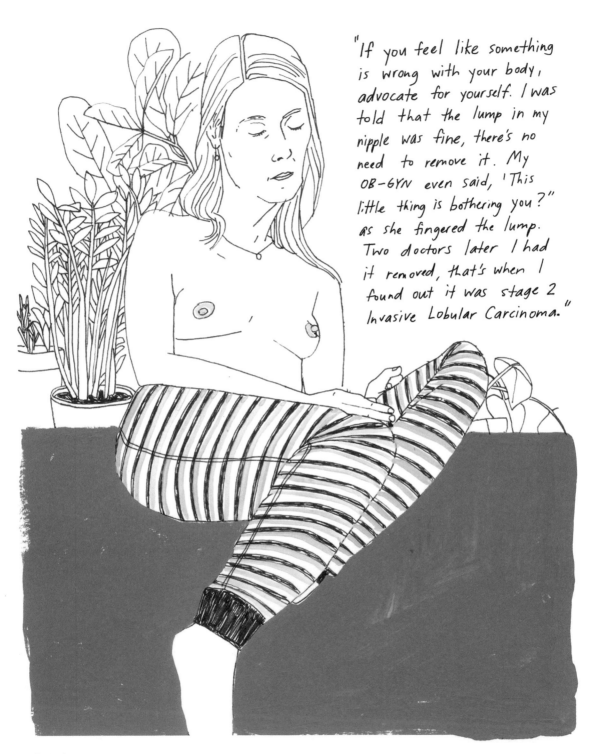

"If you feel like something is wrong with your body, advocate for yourself. I was told that the lump in my nipple was fine, there's no need to remove it. My OB-GYN even said, 'This little thing is bothering you?" as she fingered the lump. Two doctors later I had it removed, that's when I found out it was stage 2 Invasive Lobular Carcinoma."

Julia Rothman

I made up a joke about my breasts recently: *My breast size is the same as my blood group—it's A negative.*

Yes, I barely fill an A cup. And sometimes I feel bad about it. When I see pretty erotic pictures of beautiful women with nice breasts (*what does underboob feel like?*), I wish I had that. The media is full of pictures of women with round breasts. I have been feeling bad about my triangular shape for *so long*. I still do. When I wear a sweater, you can barely see them.

At the same time, my style ranges from feminine to very masculine, and I wouldn't like my masculine style with bigger breasts—I wouldn't like it on me, personally. So that's why I kind of accept my boobs. At the same time, maybe the lack of breast fuels my love for "manly" clothes.

Another thing about my breasts is that they're covered in birthmarks. I used to think, when I was ten, that they were really ugly. **Now I like them better—they kinda fill up the emptiness.** I sent a guy a nude once and he said my birthmarks were pretty, so I guess they are. *And yet* my breasts are so small that I don't need support unless I do physical activities. So I don't even need a bra, but society tells me I do.

I've tried nipple covers; they don't work on me. Those shits cost a lot of money, and they don't even work. Is it because my breasts are too triangular and there's not enough space to stick to? Are my nipples too big? Nipples are considered weird, but go outside wearing a bra and brainless young dudes will yell at you, "I can see your bra!"

Going braless is so much fun, but I usually don't have the courage to do it. I love it when I feel my soft breasts and gently squeeze them, circling around my nipples with my fingers and feeling how perfectly smooth they are. Bras are a nuisance. I own a lot of pretty bralettes, though—and one push-up. The push-up makes me crazy uncomfortable, but I need it for a certain dress that has more breast space than required for me. I also have a really large torso, which makes bra shopping an adventure. *Medium* is waaaay too big for my small whatevers, and *Small* barely fits around my ribs. I basically have all the curves except for breasts. Where is the logic? Unfair.

Of all the guys I've had sex with in my life, the smallest guy (five-foot-three) had the biggest penis, and the biggest guy (six-foot-three) had the smallest penis. So clearly you can judge an actual book by its beautiful cover, but don't judge a dude by his size!

Anyway, both sexual experiences were disappointing. The small-guy-big-penis hurt—it felt like he was poking my spine! Seriously, I felt that sex in my back. He was a boyfriend, so we settled into having incredibly slow sex, where he would inch in and then barely move around. We'd just lie there, him inside me and still. I'd breathe deeply and try to enjoy it.

The big guy-small penis was in all ways the opposite experience. He was an unexpected hook-up, a casual date who ended up in my bedroom. He whispered to me as we undressed, "Before we have sex right now, promise me that we'll have it again—that this won't be the last time." I thought it a bit odd, but I took it to mean he was interested in really building a relationship, which sounded nice! And then: sex apparently happened. I did not even realize he was inside me, but he began thrusting faster and faster, our pubic bones banging. Aha—*this* was the reason he'd attempted a pre-sex pact! **Clearly he'd suffered too many post-sex dismissals. And I became his next.**

I'm now married, and my husband's penis fits me perfectly. It took me a while to realize that the *bigger is better* cliché is just patriarchal, media-projected, macho bullshit. The best is the one that fits just right.

One time I slept with a guy who I later realized had no legs and just one hand. It was in a bar in Paris, a bar with a back room. There was a hot Brazilian and I was very attracted to him physically. He had a beautiful face. We started making out. I had been drinking for eight to ten hours at that point. He happened to put his large Brazilian penis in me, and we were going to town. I think I may have been up against a wall or something—it was a bit of a dank cave.

I remember he was behind me, and when I reached back to grab his arms I felt he had a stump on one arm. I had this moment where my brain flickered to complete sobriety, and I was like, *Oh my god, what is going on?* But it felt so good, I was like, "Fuck it!" (Literally!) "Keep going!"

I found him on Scruff the next day, and when I tapped through his naked photos it turned out both his legs were prosthetics. I didn't know because he was wearing jeans. I don't know what had happened in his life. The sex was amazing, though. And it really made me rethink how judgmental I am about my choices of who I have sex with. Usually it's so physically based. But this guy had a huge dick, and the sex was amazing. It was fine that he had no legs.

I saw him again in Paris several months later, and I knew what I was in for. I was much less drunk, and I thought, *I remember that dick, and I'm going for it. Let's do it!*

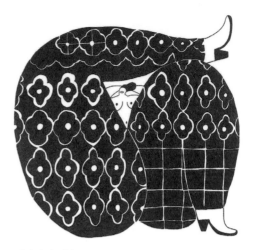

Atieh Sohrabi

When I was thirty-five, I found out I had breast cancer and had a double mastectomy because, fuck it, who needs 'em? **But as it turns out, they were more useful than I had thought when it came to feeling like a sexual being and like a woman.** Now, where my breasts used to be, I have two rock-hard implants that feel like overfilled water balloons—well, actually they don't feel like anything, because they're completely numb.

Now I wear a shirt when I have sex with my husband and won't let him touch my "breasts" because I have no sensation there and because it just reminds me of cancer, which kind of kills the mood.

I never liked my breasts. I thought they were way too big, so I'd try to hide them. **I met a lot of guys, but I felt that 90 percent of the time they were with me for my body, and that made me feel more and more uncomfortable about it.** Then when I was sixteen, I met my actual boyfriend, and within the first month I asked him, "If I didn't have these breasts and this body, would you love me?"

He was like, "Ummmm—no," and I felt sad, but then he hugged me and whispered in my ear, "You have an amazing body, and you should be so proud of it." That helped me a little, and I tried to like it and feel better about my boobs.

Years later I was hanging out without a bra on, and I was playing with my boobs while watching some movie. I squeezed them and it felt like I had a lemon—a big one—inside each one. I was scared as hell. I looked on the internet, asked friends, told my mom, and for the first time in my life I was so afraid to lose them. I went to the doctor, and they told me I have fibrocystic breasts. Since then I love them a lot.

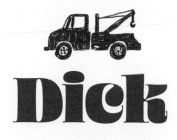

Dick

by J. COLIN HUERTER

Five or so years ago, as I was reading what seemed to be a perfectly forgettable interview with Oliver Stone, the American filmmaker, a series of intensely sexual images flashed through my mind. I suppose it's fair to call them memories now, though I hadn't realized what they were then, and trailing just after, a sudden dissipation of a long-held feeling of shame. I promise you it's not hyperbole to say it felt like an exorcism had taken place. Sitting alone at my kitchen table, where my computer was set up and I had been reading, I started crying, which eventually turned into sobbing. The waterworks lasted for nearly an hour. I was thirty-five.

Stone the provocateur was musing on his childhood—his troubled relationship with his father, his time as a soldier in Vietnam, and the like. Every few answers he'd throw in something particularly lewd, or purposely offensive, simply to keep the mood of the interview antagonistic. I could tell he wasn't happy answering the questions about his new film and preferred to change the format into a quasi–therapy session.

And yet, amid all his bluster, he said more or less the following: "My father bought me a whore for my thirteenth birthday. We were in Rome. Just he and I. I don't know where my mother was. At dinner one night, the bottles of wine kept coming. When it was time for my present, he said he had a surprise for me: 'I'm taking you to a cat house.' We were walking past the Pantheon when he explained to me he wanted to make sure my cherry was taken by a pro. He said, 'Most guys fall in love with the first skirt that spreads her legs for him.' He wanted to make sure the same thing didn't happen to me."

I had a similar experience.

Mine came a year earlier. I was twelve back then, the summer between seventh and eighth grade. But my father wasn't the one who paid for me. That was done by someone trying to take my father's place. His name was Dan, or Dave, or Dale, or Dick. Let's call him Dick.

My parents were in the middle of their divorce, and Dick and my mother were dating, or fucking, or just hanging around enough to confuse the hell out of me and my three younger siblings.

Dick worked on my mother's acreage. My mother ran a bed-and-breakfast in western Iowa, about thirty minutes from Omaha, which is where I lived during the week with my dad.

I'd spend most weekends with her. I'm sure to her I seemed lazy. I didn't like to mow the grounds, or weed the garden, or spend time outside hiking or anything active like that. One of my sisters had a horse, Bikini Beach, and she would saddle her up and ride down the lane to get the mail. I preferred to watch TV, talk on the phone, do my homework, and read. I knew my mother was worried about me. She thought I was sickly. I was pudgy and howled for days when she bought the cheap ice cream.

But whenever Dick was around, I'd close my book, find my work gloves, and tag along. Unlike my father, who was a doctor, a golfer, and an avid lover of poetry and modern art, Dick would drive piles into the ground for the new fence. He'd pour concrete for the dance floor in the old red barn. He'd cut down the dead trees in the windbreak west of the house. While working, he'd tell me about dry-humping his English teacher during his senior prom and fingering his second cousin, Karen, on a paddleboat at the zoo. He'd ask me, "Have you ever had your pecker kissed yet, or yanked?" I don't remember if I told him I had or I hadn't.

Dick was in his late twenties, strong as could be, with a long mustache that made him look like a villain from the *Street Fighter* video game. He'd wrestled in college, then spent two years on the rodeo circuit before a bull stepped on his hip and shattered it.

Most of the time I tried not to make any mistakes and to keep him happy. I'd seen him kick a dog so hard that it died on the spot. I didn't think he'd ever hit me like that, but I also didn't want to find out.

During that summer, a curious thing happened: the more we worked together, the more he began to see me as not quite as much of a fuckup as I thought myself to be. If I could handle the Weedwacker without breaking it, and the chain saw without slicing off my fingers or my pecker, then he supposed I could drive his new pickup through the fields over to his father's farm, about three miles as the crow flies, hook up the skid loader, and haul it back so we could fill the sand for the volleyball court.

One afternoon, Dick and I were in Council Bluffs to run some errands. We had to stop by Menards to pick up some nails for the pneumatic air gun; then he wanted to swing by an auto shop to see if they'd put the new engine in his Camaro yet.

As we were pulling into the parking lot, he turned to me and said, "Shelia's here—it's your lucky day."

No more than five minutes later I was climbing up into the cab of the tow truck in the shaded alley behind the shop. A few moments before, Dick had been laughing and teasing Shelia and me, calling us lovebirds, calling us the perfect match, hooting and shooing us along. Right in front of me, in front of all of us, he gave her twenty bucks and told her she'd get another twenty once she was finished. "Take a look at him," he said, pointing at me. "The automatic car wash lasts longer than he will."

Shelia was a black woman, thin, with a soft voice and a sour smell. She wore cutoff shorts, flip-flops, and a pink T-shirt with some large yellow logo on it. I remember the seats in the cab being too hot to sit on. It was the middle of an August afternoon. From the bag at her feet she pulled out a large beach towel and smoothed it out for us along the bench seats. It hit me then—she was on her way to the pool that day. She leaned over me and rolled down the window, then said something about getting the keys so we could turn the engine on and get some air going. But just as she did, I looked in the side-view mirror to my right and saw Dick and some of the other grease monkeys huddled together behind us. We heard them laugh and Dick say, "She's doing it. She's going to kiss his pecker!"

I'm pretty sure she asked how old I was. If she did, I didn't answer. She had to know I didn't have my driver's license, but did she know I wasn't even in high school yet? I'm sure I didn't ask her her age. She could have been anywhere between twenty and forty.

Now that I no longer carry around the shame about it, as I had for all those years; now that I know that other fathers (and father figures) have done the same thing to other small boys as a rite of passage; now that I can situate myself on some kind of spectrum, with child abuse on one side and sexual perversion on the other, I can more freely remember the erotic feeling of her hot hand against my stomach as she lifted up my shirt and began to unzip my jeans. I wasn't hard. Shelia said, "It's all right," then took out her left breast and placed my hand on it. With that, I became hard enough for her to slip the condom on.

Five years have passed since that series of images flashed through my mind and gave me my final release. All of them have returned to where they came, along with my shame. All of them except for the image of her black hair lying over my entire lap, like some wig of pubic hair.

FIRST TIMES

SHAINA There's so much buildup, so much anxiety and anticipation about losing your virginity.

JULIA And then you do it and you're like, that's *it*?

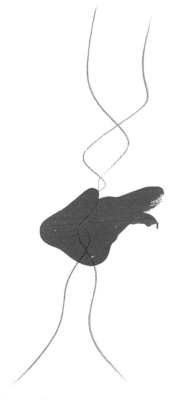

Roman Muradov

Growing up, I was conditioned to regard an unwed pregnancy as the worst possible outcome of premarital sex. **Of course, even nineteen years of fearmongering didn't stop me from losing my virginity during my freshman year of college to my boyfriend of six months.**

It was the morning after a fantastic, low-key Valentine's Day date that involved Thai food and reggae. We were lying in my lofted-too-close-to-the-ceiling-bed when I said, "Let's have sex."

His eyes widened: "Really?"

"Yeah, I want to."

He decamped to retrieve a condom. Then we took off our clothes and began making out. He unwrapped the condom, put it on, and eased inside me. I looped my arms under his and gripped his shoulders as he pushed and pulled, gently, in and out of me. Having him inside me felt weird, but not unpleasant—I don't know what my face was doing, but it prompted him to ask if I was okay—and ended pretty quickly. Sweat beaded along his brow and above his lips. His face was beautiful, his eyes closed, and his mouth formed into a giddy grin.

"Hey?"

"Hey." I kissed him and ran my hands through his hair as he withdrew and slid down next to me on the bed.

The condom had broken.

I shifted into panic immediately. My boyfriend—bless him—calmly tried to remind me about the morning-after pill. So we picked up Plan B from the pharmacy, along with some chocolate milk and a seventy-two count box of condoms—but a different brand!

The first time I had
sex was in the back
seat of my father's
car, and the woman
said she'd always imagined
the first time would
be on a bed of roses.
She laughed and I
laughed and we
laughed. And in my
head I thought:
This relationship won't
last long.

It was both of our first times and we were definitely too young. You couldn't have told us that then, but we were. We had met at church and went to different schools, so church events and Facebook messaging was the only way we communicated. We had started with just making out, sexting, and so on, and finally we devised a plan to go all the way.

During the forty-five minutes of Sunday school, she would leave her class and sneak to the women's restroom. I would then leave *my* Sunday school class and sneak to the men's restroom. **Each of those bathrooms had an unlocked door leading to a stairway, and this stairway led to the men's and women's side of the baptistery.** The two were connected by the large tub where the baptisms would happen. We knew it would be empty, so when I got up there I softly crossed the tub to the women's side, a thin curtain the only thing keeping me from being seen by the entire church sanctuary.

When I got to her side, we took each other's virginity on the threadbare blue carpet, and it definitely didn't take the forty-five minutes we had allotted. In what was probably fifteen minutes from when we left, we were both back in our respective classes.

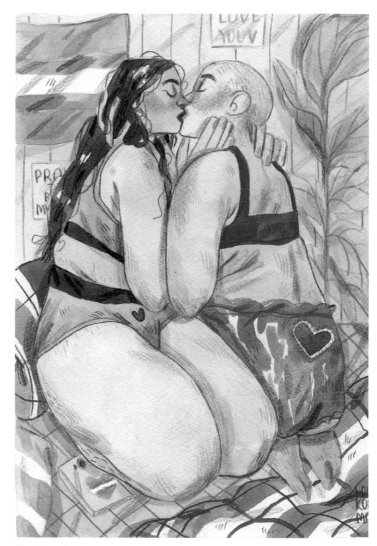

Eleni Koumi

Both being from conservative evangelical families, we didn't know much about birth control or sex in general, so no contraception was used. Even if we had wanted to, we had no way of getting any: neither of us was old enough to drive at the time, and our Deep South schools taught abstinence and provided no contraceptives.

Later, after she and I had broken up, I used the same place for the first guy I ever had intercourse with. I was a little older, a little wiser, and a lot more pleased at the sacrilege of us "sodomizing" each other in that evangelical church.

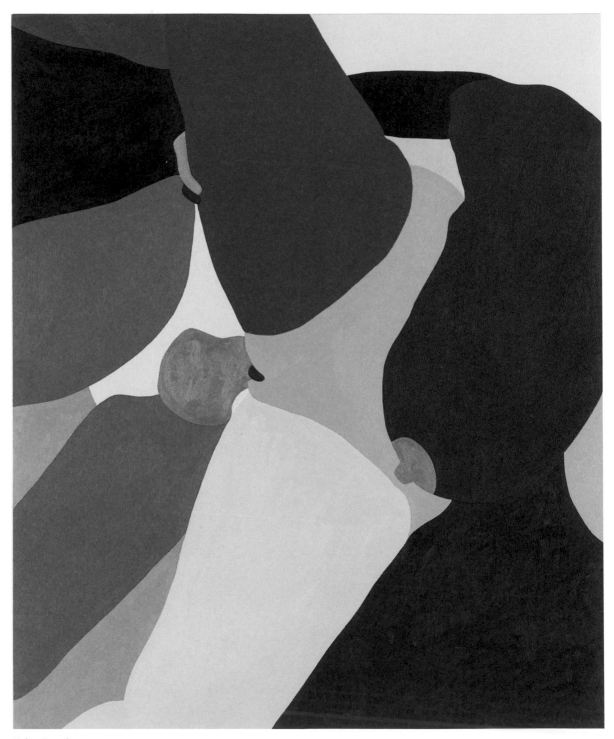

Helen Beard

EVERY

My first time was really, really good. Of all my friends, I was the "late guy"; I was nineteen. It was Southern California. I went on a date with this girl and she took me home. **She really took control of the situation because I didn't know what I was doing.** She was on top of me. When I came, she whispered in my ear, "Wasn't that amazing? It feels like your brain is floating on champagne bubbles." And it really did.

My first time I was really lucky. We were both virgins and I was fifteen. We had done everything, make-out wise. **We had been regularly going to third base.** My parents were going out of town and I invited her to stay at my house. My whole fear was that it would hurt for her. But then if I was already sticking four fingers in her, I thought, my dick's not that big. I went in slowly. She said, "This feels really good." I came in probably sixty seconds. I was so scared of her getting pregnant that we had ten condoms lined up, just in case. The greatest thing about it is that she said, "Do it again—I want more." Over the next few days, all we wanted to do was have sex. It felt powerful.

I was around twelve or thirteen when I learned about sex by having my first relationship. **It was with my uncle.** It was good. It was my mom's brother. It went on for two or three years.

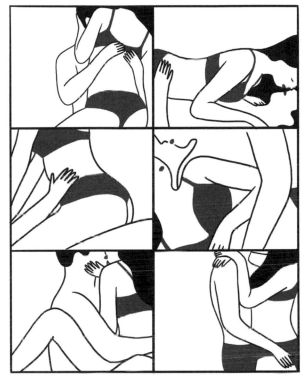

Agathe Sorlet

I was twenty-two the first time I had sex—which felt ancient at the time. I had been seeing my boyfriend, Sebastian, for several months. Because I was well into my twenties, I assumed I wouldn't bleed. I had read that young women often break their hymens by playing sports, wearing tampons—whatever. So I was shocked when I bled like the dickens!

Here's what I remember vividly, all these years later: afterward, he gently, gently carried me to the shower. He gently, gently set me down and ran the shower and brought me a clean white towel and wrapped me up. And that was the best possible lesson I could have learned: **sometimes it's not the sex that matters, but the care and kindness and reverence with which someone treats your body.**

I was fifteen and dating a super-popular senior at our high school. His name was "Jake Mettle" (name changed for privacy) and he drove a '66 blue Mustang. He had blond hair and bright blue eyes and always smelled good, even though he worked at the local gas station. He drove me to school daily, and I felt supercool.

I thought I needed to sleep with him to keep him dating me, so one night we went down to the beach to make out. It was cold but his breath was husky and warm; he'd had a beer earlier, which I could taste. We were lying on a blanket in the sand and decided to go all the way. It was fast, awkward, and sandy—I don't think he ever really got it in, but I do remember going home with sand in my underpants. I clearly didn't know what I was doing—and he didn't want to bother to take the time to show me.

The next day, he ignored me at school. I was mortified. To make the situation even more amazing, my best friend suddenly decided I might be pregnant and called my mother to tell her what had happened. I got dragged to the gynecologist, who proceeded to inform my mother that my hymen hadn't even been broken, so nothing to worry about. A humiliating yet memorable way to lose my virginity, for sure.

My second time was about a year later. I was in Mexico with my family. I was super-drunk at the resort we were staying at and met a cute guy who seemed really into me from my intoxicated perspective. I was sixteen and eager to prove that I could figure this sex thing out. We went to his room, and ended up outside on his balcony, so as not to wake his roommate. Try number two still didn't really get it, and the next day when I went to find him at the pool he literally waved me away. Despite my frequent fantasies and masturbation, I thought I simply might not be destined to be a sexual person after all, so I decided to focus on other things.

Third time really is a charm. I put off having sex again until college; funny enough, I ended up at an all-women's school. My roommate, Jamie, had a long, lanky body with short blond hair. Not really my type, but her laugh...I had never been with a woman before, despite some crushes, but one night we had gone to a party and I was quite tipsy. I was in my bed and she asked if she could crawl in. The room was spinning and her hands began to wander across my body. I could finally feel the want. Her tongue was velvet and warm, and I suddenly knew what to do. We explored each other until early dawn, lying entangled, dozing in and out of wakefulness. She even talked to me the next day, and the day after that. **We spent a year as roommates and lovers, then went our separate ways. But I am grateful she finally showed me how to do it.**

We planned the day. He was seventeen and I was sixteen. We both wanted to know what "real" sex felt like. He was my boyfriend for exactly three months of my senior year. We decided that two months of being boyfriend-girlfriend was too short, but three was okay. I bought new underwear and painted my nails.

On the chosen day, we met at his house while his parents were at work. He lit two candles and put them on the table. Classic Queen was playing in the background. We closed the curtains to hide the sun. And we made out on his twin bed like we usually did. My crotch felt so hot, like it was burning. He asked me if I was sure. I said yes and he slid inside me. I felt full. The fullness traveled through my body. Our bare chests touched. As he pushed inside me, my body felt different than ever before, like he was really in me. He kissed my neck and lips. A few times asked me if I was okay. And I felt amazing. It lasted two songs.

There was more wetness and more warmth than I was used to. I didn't realize that it would pour out of me when I stood up. But I liked the feeling that a part of him was still there. I wanted to cry because I was so relieved, but I didn't because I thought I might scare him. His mom was on her way home from work and I had to leave fast. I took the bus home. I wondered if anyone could tell. I felt so different.

When he called me that night, I told him I wanted more. We skipped classes and had a ton of sex for the next few months. We had sex every time we saw each other. It's all we would do when we were together. I started missing other stuff, like watching movies and just talking, but I didn't tell him. I got into my dream college and he got rejected from the same one. He was depressed. I was getting excited for the new chapter of my life but I felt guilty talking about it. We decided to end things before college, and we didn't talk for the whole summer.

College was different. People went crazy—everyone was having sex with guys at frat parties when they were drunk and high. Sometimes I got close, but it seemed gross. I missed my boyfriend. Against my roommate's advice, one Friday night I took a two-hour Greyhound bus ride to his college and showed up unexpectedly at his dorm. I put on my favorite jeans, a black tank top, and some makeup. I felt sexy. I didn't even know if he was there and I didn't have a plan. I just wanted to see him. He was in the common room, hanging out with his friends. He was surprised and seemed super-happy. He introduced me to his friends and we told stories all night. But mostly we had heaps of sex.

I didn't want to leave and I missed all my classes on Monday. He promised he would call and visit me too, but he didn't. I never saw him again.

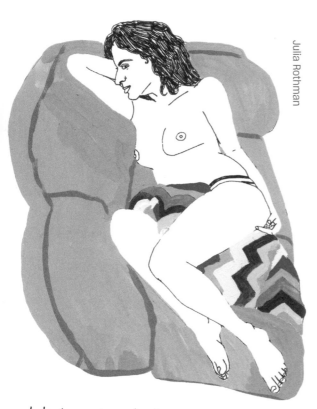

Julia Rothman

I lost my virginity kind of late. I was waiting until I was in love. I loved him as a person but I don't think I was actually in love with him. But I had just turned 21, was studying abroad in London and was ready to lose the "virgin" label and do this thing that it seemed like everyone around me had already been doing for years. We were in Scotland (he was Scottish). So there was that accent, and those hills, and you kind of couldn't beat that for a first time. Except his dog watching us. I could have lost that.

I was a late bloomer for a few different sexual milestones, one being the much-celebrated penis-fully-inside-vagina. The first time I tried it there was a slight pinch as my hymen broke, followed immediately by a bunch more pain as his penis pushed about an inch farther in. I stopped us. We chilled. **I sat on my ankle and let the blood collect in the hollow above my heel.**

I was freaked out by how much it hurt, and the trust issue was already a little weird. (He would boast that I was the fifth girl whose virginity he had taken, and I found that to be the opposite of comforting.) We broke up because I kept not wanting to try again.

Next boyfriend down the line, we tried. Got to the same point minus the pinch, but again a lot of pain. We stopped, frozen in position, and took a breather and chatted. A minute or so later, my boyfriend informed me, wide-eyed, "You have a penis inside you," bewildered that this was something that needed to be said out loud. He was absolutely right—I did now have a penis inside me!

I realized it had been a matter of the muscles tensing at the base of my pelvis, and they hurt when pushed against. Those muscles had relaxed while we chatted, letting him slide inside so easily I hadn't even felt it.

Having carried around this dread of pain and this confusion about my body for some time, I howled with laughter. My boyfriend, understandably, immediately lost his boner. But we tried again as soon as it was phallically feasible, and had a bunch more penis-fully-in-vagina sex—henceforth pain-free.

In 2016 was the first time I ever made love. I lost my virginity. I met this beautiful French woman in the park. I was playing soccer with my friends, and we were talking in French. **She walked over and said, "You're a French guy?"** That was the icebreaker introduction. She came here from France to get her tooth fixed. She is older. We connected. She likes to dance. I'm a dancer. One day she took me to a club to hang out. We had drinks. We hung out. I went to her house. I cleaned it. I fixed things. I cooked for her. Then we made love. Every time she comes to this country, she wants to hang out. She is double my age. When I met her I was twenty-six and she was fifty. I don't date otherwise. I love her, but I can't stay with her, because one day I will marry a woman who can give birth.

When I was seventeen, I briefly dated a guy in my class. It was hard to get privacy to do anything intimate. As a result, our first sexual experience took place in a tree house in a local park. It was late in the evening during winter, so no kids were about! We kissed and he fingered me and went down on me. Considering our lack of experience, it felt better than I thought it would. **Unfortunately, we were abruptly interrupted by two men climbing up the ladder.** I quickly pulled up my underwear and tights, and we sat there pretending to have a conversation. The builders politely smiled at us and walked through to the other side of the tree house to fix a swing. I was horrendously embarrassed. After they left, we left too; it was getting cold and the mood had died.

The guy and I broke up not long after. I thought that we would be able to get on afterward, but I think it affected him worse. I decided the dislike was mutual when he eventually called me a slut behind my back. However, I still remember that tree-house incident fondly.

We hadn't been dating that long. We were at his house after school. **We ended up having sex on his bed, with his mom in the living room.** It was my first time. It hurt bad, but I acted like it was fantastic. He kissed me too much. I couldn't get a breath the whole time. I don't think he was all that big, but it sure felt like I was dying. His mom knocked on the door while we were in the middle of it all. She ended up opening the door just as he slid off me and lay beside me with the blankets over us. She just asked what he wanted to eat. I know she knew what we were doing, but she chose to ignore it.

He didn't wear a condom, and I told him I wasn't a virgin. He learned the truth the second his mom shut the door and he pulled off the covers: blood everywhere. Hello, hymen! All over his penis, all over his bed. I shot up with embarrassment, pulled my white jean shorts back on, and got blood all over them. Left in a hurry.

He was very confused. So was I. I didn't know it at the time, but I had endometriosis and it caused way more bleeding than was considered normal. I walked out that front door with his mom facing my bloody ass with no fucks. We dated for three years. She always seemed to like me, but none of us ever talked about that day. And she was the type of mom that did her seventeen-year-old son's laundry, so I can only imagine what she thought.

When he broke up with me years later because I was "too emotional," I felt a sense of pride knowing I had ruined his mattress all that time ago. Ha!

By the Sidewalk: A Memory

by FARIHA RÓISÍN

It happens for everyone in different ways.

Mine happened on the side of the sidewalk in a park just by the entrance of the Sydney Botanical Gardens. I was wedged between the Sydney Opera House and the Sydney Harbor Bridge—floating on a side angle as I pulled down the pants of my then-boyfriend. Sloping, we lost our virginity to each other on a hillside. Barnacles and dirt our bed for the five minutes it took for me to fidget my vagina onto his body scrunched up by a tree.

We were both nervous. His pants, ugly black slacks like a bank teller's, were rolled down to his ankles—and when I finally found it, his penis looked like a hairy little elephant's trunk, all shrunken and shy. I wanted to laugh—and scream. I did neither. Instead, I forced myself into a sexual mood. *Perform, bitch,* I repeated in my head, nervously rattling a sex chant to myself. This was the best chance we were going to get. The mood was just right. I had made an elaborate excuse to be out for the night, at least till, like, 10 p.m. The mood was alriiiighhhht.

And damn, I needed to fuck—period.

I was tired of keeping my legs closed. I had waited like a good little girl, patient. My god, I was ready. I wanted to get rammed up the side of the tree, filled in by full, passionate thrusts, my clit all juicy against his right thumb. I wanted us to come together, stained with sweat by the end of it. Instead, it was barely two inches inside me before he came. Heady, we laughed, embarrassed by our messiness.

We were both South Asians—and you know South Asian teens can't casually fuck in their parents' homes, right? A Hindu Indian and a Muslim Bangladeshi banging away all their feelings of shame? It's just not kosher. With all that surveillance? Under whose watch? Forget about it.

So outdoor, public sex became my first consensual foray into sexual activity. I was in my late teens, bright and deeply self-hating. I hated my body, my god—I hated it all. My skin, so sallow and puckered—my knees always ashy. My body felt so masculine to me. I thought I was slovenly, caked in fat like a cast-iron pan with a residue of old grease.

And, listen, I wasn't one of those thick girls with big titties, a small waist, and a fat ass. No, I had two of those things—disproportionate—like I was not (at all) made in God's image. Instead (to me, and seemingly *only me*) I was a visual atrocity, a bastardized version of what an attractive young girl oughta be.

So this sense of wanting, of being seen by someone who acutely understood your cultural dimensions, filled a gnawing gap. As if we both saw the other, mirrored.

We were attracted to how similar we were, how we hated ourselves in the same ways. We fucked to close the void of whiteness—the shame of not being white—as if we were each other's chance at survival. In sex we could forget about the myths we'd been fed of our bodies, of the lies we'd been told about our desirability (or lack thereof). We came together to forgive ourselves of our ugliness. We fucked away the pain.

It was deep.

For months we fucked in public bathrooms, dark alleys, in the back seat and in dried-up bushes. As an unassuming Muslim girl—and a relatively nonrebellious one at that—I learned how to sneak out of the house with ceaseless effort. I was impressed by myself; even my CIA agent of an insomniac mother never found out. So he and I became the neighborhood fuck unit, and it felt weirdly freeing. Like, for the first time I was living my life.

Once—and only once—we "made love" (underwhelmingly) in his childhood room. He kept his white undershirt on, his skin flabby underneath it from all the weight he had recently lost. Surrounding us were posters of Mafia movies: *Goodfellas,* all three *Godfathers,* a *Scarface* poster of Pacino on a throne. It made sense that he looked up to these old, skeezy, dim-witted Italian patriarchs; he was learning misogyny fast. His sex-making played into a masculinity that was so very performative. But what is gender, if anything?

After a while, I knew there was something wrong. Our fucking had grown erratic; we were losing the excitement of losing our collective virginhood to one another. I knew that my body had begun to bore him, I could see his entitlement to it. Like that meme with the white kid's vein throbbing out of his head—spontaneous human combustion. When masculinity becomes toxic, you're doing it wrong, babe.

He eventually told me that he wanted "more" (code: *not you*). He wanted "someone more statuesque" (read: *beautiful, model;* read: *white*). I felt ashamed that I wasn't any of those things. I began to believe that this was a failure on my part.

There's a time, especially if you come from where I came from (where sexuality is governed, tamed, and watched), when you have to start learning how to pace yourself when you launch into sex. But I didn't know! I was way too young to know how to stop the red flame of seduction in my body. So after we broke up...I became a nympho.

I wasn't expecting it either.

I told myself Allah would forgive me as I masturbated to a vibrating duck. Saying Surah Al Fatihah later, crying that I was losing my good

Muslim self. I started to lust after dripping pussies and thick, tight thighs, becoming a lesbian in hiding and then flip-flopping back to men like a pendulum. I wanted it all. But, most importantly, I wanted to disintegrate into dust as I got fucked and stayed fucked by all the dildos, tongues, and dicks that would have me.

I started to lose my faith in the madness. It's as if because I'd had my desire on a leash for so long, by the time I accepted it I was bungee jumping into the future. I was lit with passion, with verve, with a newfound identity. For the first time, I felt like I wasn't hiding. I wanted to be my fully sexual self: a ravenous monster.

But this journey, reader, was a long one. So long that I'm still on it. Still learning how to forgive myself for my rapturous need to be filled with cum, like I'm constantly a drug addict who needs a hit. Sometimes it feels devastating.

It took me a while to come back to faith. To understand that Allah was there all along. That I could be myself in all of its complications, but that despite all the hardship, I knew one thing to be true: I couldn't exist *without* Islam. It was my entire metric of being human.

There's a composition to a Muslim woman. Whether we are fully veiled in a burqa or a niqab—or wearing Nike trainers and sweats, miniskirts and stripper heels—we've learned how to move past the stereotypes people will have of us. Faceless, desireless, one-dimensional, lacking depth. We defy stereotypes every goddamn day!

I wish I had understood that truth when the first person I ever fucked dumped me like a fake Gucci handbag at a Salvation Army. I wish I had someone tell me that I should slow down, that I should like myself, that I don't need to prove anything to anybody—and least of all to prove it with sex. That my body will grow on me in ways I never thought possible, that I don't have to punish it so hard. I wish someone had told me that white girls will say some shit but really they want to be you in private. I wish I had been reminded earlier that I won't have my body forever, that I'm lucky to have it. I should cherish it, that things will one day make sense. I wish I'd known sooner that the sexual shame will be rooted in something sinister, memories that I had put away, but that that's my journey and that I should learn to forgive myself. That I should learn to find myself beautiful—and enjoy the beauty of other South Asian women as well.

There's a part of me that deeply hates the beginning of all this.

I can still see the moonlight lining the streets, sheets of light from the streetlamp pour through like passages shadowing where we lie, sloping.

Under the tree we smile at each other, eager to lose the burden of virginity. But it's rushed, somewhat forced. In the years since, it's taught me bad sexual habits and reinforced a lack of boundaries. But at the end of the day, I'm glad it happened. I'm mainly happy with the results. Sure, it lacked romance and true care in the moment...but I guess my only solace is that it happens for everyone in different ways.

RELIGION

JULIA Whenever I was dating someone, my grandma would ask, "Is he Jewish?" And I would say no. And my grandma would say, "Well, you're not getting married yet."

SHAINA I grew up Jewish, and when I got married to my husband, Chris, who grew up Irish Catholic, we were like, *Let's have someone marry us who isn't Catholic or Jewish.* So we asked our friend Ruby. Well, at the ceremony the first words out of her mouth were, "Jesus, bless this union." Both Chris and I were shocked, but we just went along with it.

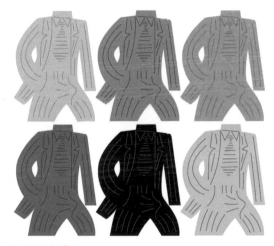

Farshid Shafiey

I'm a cis-het woman who grew up with extremely conservative Christian Asian parents who were very much against sex before marriage. So when I began dating in high school and college, I knew that sex wasn't something I could talk to my parents about—I had a bevy of smart, cool friends and the internet for that. Then in college my mom found out that I had gone on a weekend trip with my boyfriend, and she was furious—just so incredibly angry—because she knew it meant that I'd had sex. **I was twenty-one at the time, but that call with my mom unhinged me, and I instantly lied, saying nothing had happened.** I was devastated thinking she'd never see me the same way again, but later she gave me a call and told me that she loved me no matter what and that I was an adult and she trusted me.

I think I learned that while there are things I'd rather not bring up with my parents because it would cause them distress, and they'd probably rather not know, I try not to lie to them anymore. I'm more sure of their love for me—and, more radically, of the things that I deserve to receive from the people I love. This includes respect for my decisions as an adult woman, even if they are not completely aligned with the choices they want me to make.

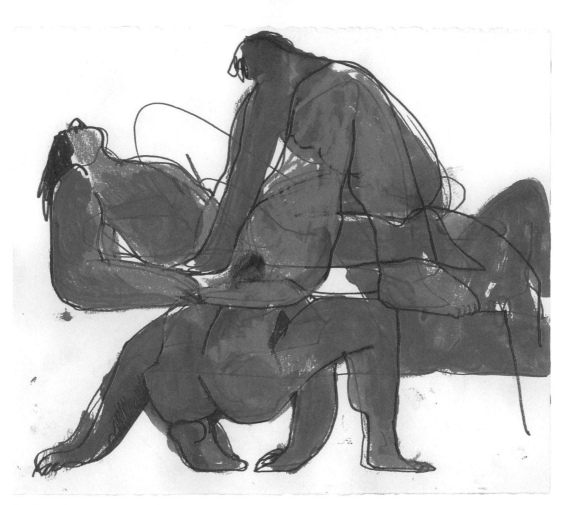

Alex Eben Meyer

In 1971 the preacher's son had just come home from Vietnam, and I screwed him in the church bathroom—we were standing up. I was eighteen years old, he was nineteen. We smoked pot afterward—in the church bathroom! It was a Baptist church in Harlem. **We were supposed to be in Sunday school class, but instead we were screwing in the bathroom.** It feels good to get that off my chest.

I never realized my mother was religious until after I revealed to her that I had had sex. She grew up in Soviet Russia, and I always assumed she had a progressive and secular stance on things. I was nineteen at the time, and while we were talking about my boyfriend I brought up that I had slept with him. She refused to speak to me for a week. She started reading old religious tracts that I didn't know she owned. I felt like some godless whore. The texts were in Old Church Slavonic.

Her views haven't stopped me, but I wish she could be happy for me. She still seems to believe that I've lost something important.

I am twenty-one now. I live in Kazakhstan. My family is religious and conservative. We never talk about sex. I am a girl. **It is considered a shame to talk to your father even about dating or love.** When I was ten or eleven, I read about masturbation on the internet. I found porn and masturbated. I felt really good but felt embarrassed. I felt that it was wrong.

As I grew older and entered high school, I became more and more religious, but I could not stop myself from masturbation. Every time I was doing it, I thought that my dead relatives were looking and that they were ashamed of me. I felt that they were watching me every time I masturbated. I felt so ashamed of myself. I thought that I was the only one like that. I thought a good Muslim girl couldn't be like this. I thought that I was a liar, a sinner. I thought I would go to hell. I fasted and prayed so God would forgive me.

When I entered university, I found different feminist pages on Instagram and read feminist books and watched feminist movies. I realized that masturbation and sex are beautiful and one should never be ashamed of them. I am a senior in university now. Now I realize how beautiful my body is. Now I know a lot about sex education and I will speak to my children openly about it in the future. I want them to feel free to ask questions on this topic and tell me about their insecurities. I will show them that sex and love are so natural and they should never be ashamed to talk about them.

I had just gotten off a flight back to NYC and was waiting for the AirTrain when I got a call from a guy I previously hooked up with. He asked to see me and told me to meet him at a train stop off the J. I still had my luggage with me and it was snowing pretty hard. He helped me trek through the snow to what I assumed was his place. Turns out where we were headed to was his grandma's apartment. **I awkwardly met his grandma, who was a practicing Catholic Dominican woman who had rosary beads and a life-size Jesus statue in her living room.** She later went to her room to take a nap.

At one point I remember going to use the bathroom and saw that I was spotting, which I took as a sign from Jesus. When I walked out, the guy was in the kitchen and I met him there. He started to kiss me and tried to hook up. First, I thought about how his grandma was less than 100 feet away in her small New York apartment bedroom. Second, I thought about how my period was starting, and third I thought about the judgment I would receive from life-size Jesus. We inevitably hooked up in the kitchen—doggy-style, on the floor. When he finished, I saw that a spot of my period blood had stained his white shirt.

I am from a very conservative and Catholic part of Mexico. It really affected me the way we look at sex: basically we do not have any information or education. **It is all about abstinence—that's the only thing they tell you.** When I was in my early twenties, I realized I shouldn't be ashamed of it; it's normal to have sex. I then tried to inform myself before having sex, but the doctor I consulted made me feel horrible. She told me that I was going to get an STD and get super-sick. She told me that I needed to think about it. She asked me: "Do you really want to have sex?"

I finally found the right doctor to get informed, and I found the person I wanted to have sex with. It was not great, but I did it. It was my decision, and I felt great about it. When I moved to the UK, I realized how much of a stigma sex is in my home country. The worst part is that there are so many issues around sex back in Mexico because of the lack of sex education. It is very frustrating to realize how these ideas affect my family and friends, teenage pregnancies, and abuse. I hope that one day we will talk and learn more openly about sex. I believe it could be a big difference. It is normal to have sex—you should enjoy it, and it should not be a stigma.

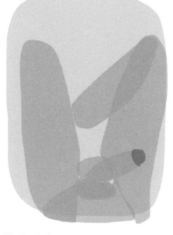

Tio Cuchillos

I grew up kind of religious, but not super-religious. **When I was young I wanted to save myself for marriage, but just because I'm a romantic.** It seemed so romantic. My mom saved herself for marriage, and my parents love each other so much, and I was like, *I want that!* But then I got into sex, and I was like, *Never mind!*

I grew up in a strict, religious household, which forbade me to have sex before marriage. I dated my first boyfriend (who had already had plenty of sexual experience) at age eighteen. In an effort to respect my boundaries, we only made out—and sometimes he would kiss my breasts. One time during a make-out session while we were both fully clothed, he humped my vagina so hard that he ejaculated in his jeans. It was like three pumps? I was bewildered and disgusted, but after he went to change his pants, he came back and told me he loved me. I guess it felt good for him. Ten years later, I've since gotten married to another guy, also sexually experienced—but, contrary to my first boyfriend, my husband is a gem (and yes, I waited until we were married to have sex). We enjoy a healthy sex life, but we make sure I'm in on the enjoyment, too.

I learned about sex from my American girlfriend when I came to America from India. I was twenty-seven. **Before this woman, I knew only what I learned in biology class about the male organ and female organ. That's it.** My parents never had the "birds and bees" talk that you Americans have. No clue. What is bird? What is bee? What do they have to do with it? Even though in India we have the *Kama Sutra*, they don't teach you that. It's a taboo.

If you come from a conservative family like I do (my parents are priests and everything), you are raised to be with just one woman. That's it. You explore together. There were arranged marriages. I was supposed to get married. But one month before, I ran away to America.

The first time I dated a woman [here], she thought there was something wrong with me. I thought, *If I am going to have sex with this girl, I am going to marry her.* I was trying to make sure she was marriage material and all that. We were going on dates, but when it came to physical intimacy I would withdraw. I was going to get married to her. My friends said we were not good for each other, but I was trying to be with her because I saw her as my wife, so I was not going to be with anyone else.

She actually broke it off. We were engaged and going to get married in Hawaii. It was 2004.

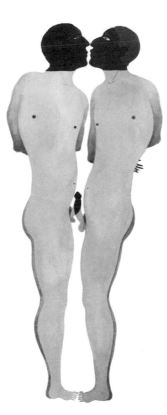

Balint Zsako

My parents refused to come, even though I was going to send tickets and everything. They said, "If you go through with this, you are not our son anymore." That pressure was on her too. She didn't want me to lose my family for her sake.

Everything happens for a reason—I believe in karma, you know. The Big Guy has big plans for me probably. I'm actually looking to become a monk.

That means no more drinking, no more partying, no more sex. Nothing. Celibacy. Everything very minimal. I understand there is more to life than going through emotions. Particularly when I see all my married friends. They did the traditional-union marriage. They had two kids. They put them through college. And still I see them hanging out with me, going to some strip clubs.

I had my first orgasm
at age twelve, smack
in the middle of an
evangelical church service.
Right there in the sanctuary!
I was just sitting there—
apparently it's called
a spontaneous orgasm. Well,
thank "God" for that, but
I don't go to church anymore.

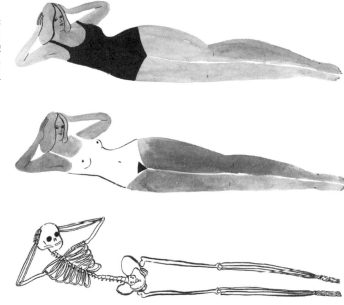

Kaye Blegvad

I honestly had no awareness of what my clit was and was confused by his attention to it (the first time I looked at my own vagina and explored it, I was twenty). My relationship to family, God, my body, my sexuality, my church, and to intimacy have not been the same since the abuse was uncovered and has seemed worse as I've pursued recovery. Talks of marriage, dating, and singleness feel constricting. I sometimes wonder if—and I despise knowing that—in ten years I may become just another sexually abused, sexually inactive (except for fantasies and masturbation) woman in my church who still feels she can't get married because she believes she is so internally broken.

No one knows how to make a place in the church for abuse/assault victims, the LGBT community, or any other individual/group with sexual questions, problems, or confidence. Support, love, and recovery often must be found outside its walls. My hope for my young church is that it will begin to acknowledge these areas where many people have gotten stuck, confused, or have escaped the church, and that it will seek to help repair those relationships and bring healing to our spiritual nature as well. Until then, "Fuck off" to the church, "Be careful" to the world, and "Shut down" to my confusing feelings seem like the safest options to live and recover between both extremes.

I've never had sex. For that matter, I've never had a boyfriend. I'm twenty one years old and just had my first make-out session this year. I am a Christian. **I'm very protective of myself sexually, but I hate feeling inexperienced.** I am naturally curious of both sexes and have desires and fantasies of each, but at times I feel like I could live with no sexual desires at all. Sexual desires tend to be very repressed in the church. I hate it because I feel like I'm not attractive to anyone, or that no one else is good enough to be attracted to. There's a lot of shame, secrecy, and high expectations, which leads to a lot of people being paralyzed in their sexuality. I don't feel free to explore mine within the church or within my religious community. I believe what the Bible says is true, but I understand and resonate with the rest of the world. I don't know how to exist when I want to keep my Christian sexual values but get out of the Christian sexual world. I'm scared to meet anyone outside a safe church circle, because I don't want to cause myself any further confusion or loss of support by becoming sexually open, promiscuous, or identifying as bisexual or lesbian.

My sexuality and spirituality are also particularly damaged because I was molested by my grandfather, a deacon in the church. He fucked with young boys and girls. He was obsessed with my clit and trying to make me feel good, even using a vibrator once without my consent.

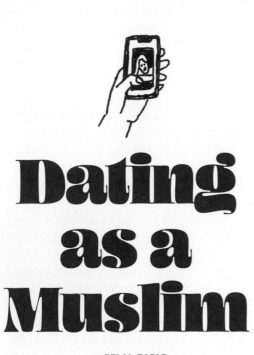

Dating as a Muslim

by **BILAL ZAFAR**

I managed to make myself the center of attention at my brother's wedding. I was "hosting" it, which wasn't that difficult to do because I'm a stand-up comedian, but working for free is always a bit annoying. It was a big, fancy event with about 300 guests, my family and I were all matching in navy, and there was a massive cake. Half the people at the wedding seemed to come up to me and jokingly say, "You're next!" like it was some sort of threat; I had to force a big laugh every time. Marriage is something that I hadn't really thought about seriously before, but all of these random family friends I was pretending to know were right: I don't have a huge family in the UK, I'm the youngest of three brothers and the only single one left, so I *am* "next."

The next morning as I was getting through some leftover wedding cake, my mother mentioned that I really should start to think about getting married. I pretended to be on a phone call and left the room, even though I didn't have a phone on me. I'm not against the idea of marriage or anything—it's something I would like to do—but talking about it with my parents has always made me cringe. Plus I could find a wife/soul mate myself, if I wanted.

Well, to be honest, I expected it to have happened by now. I'm a twenty-seven-year-old British Pakistani Muslim man; I assumed I would just meet someone at university who liked me and eventually marry her, but that was about six years ago now. Still, there's obviously plenty of people out there, but how do I actually go about this marriage thing?

I get to audition for acting roles as part of my job, and it has unexpectedly opened my eyes to how Muslims are seen—even in an industry we all consider to be "woke." When I'm going for a character with a Muslim name, he'll usually be a total idiot (which I'm surprisingly bad at playing) or something to do with a stereotype around extremism or a forced marriage—presented as inaccurately and cringe worthy as possible—with a white protagonist to save the day.

Forced marriage is a very serious issue around the world, but as a Muslim I've personally never come across it. My parents had an arranged marriage and still seem to like each other. This meant their parents introduced them to each other with marriage in mind, and it all went according to plan. That may still be a very popular way to do things among Muslims today, but as a young and (apparently) promising London-based comedian, surely I'm way too cool to have my parents set something up for me?

So I decided that dating apps were the fashionable, modern way to go.

I had tried the usual dating apps like Bumble and Tinder with no luck, so I decided to go for a slightly different approach. Going on the app store, I discovered several Muslim versions of Tinder. There were also dating apps specifically for Jewish people, for Hindus, for women who want to date bearded men, and even one exclusively for celebrities—something I might be allowed on in a year? (Maybe two?)

But for now I was focusing on Muslim Tinder-style apps called Minder and Muzmatch. The first step, as with any dating app, is to fill in some information about yourself and upload a photo that makes you look much better than you are. It started off easy:

NAME: Bilal

AGE: 27

But then things got a bit tricky. I got to PROFESSION and it didn't let me type any words in; instead there was a drop-down list with no option for *Comedian, Actor,* or even *Writer,* so I ended up typing in *Other.* It wasn't the best start. I know that artsy jobs aren't generally held in high regard among Muslims (or people in general), but the fact that this app thinks we don't even exist felt a bit harsh.

I tried my best to create an exciting little bio for myself. I thought I was all set, but there was one final thing before I could start my journey. The app asked, "How religious are you?" I wasn't expecting this level of interrogation from a dating app. I'd never been asked this question before, and I wasn't even sure what it meant. Was it asking me how good a person I think I am? It's all so subjective. I do a lot of praying when a sports team I support is playing, but I'm not sure if that counts. Again, I wasn't allowed to type in a word to answer this question; instead I was presented with a sliding scale to mark "how religious" I am. Finally deciding to put it at about halfway, I was ready to start my Mindering—and find the love of my life!

A lot like on Tinder, I got a match, but no one spoke for about thirty minutes. I spoke first: "Hi." Then I remembered this is Muslim Tinder, so I went with "Salaam." I came across plenty of nice women my age who said they were seeking marriage within a year or two. I find it amazing that anyone can plan their life so clearly: my rail pass expires in a year, and I have literally no idea what I'm going to do when that happens. I found myself having to explain that my parents are actually okay with (and sometimes even supportive of) my career choice, and not disappointed. When asked what my caste is, I got confused and answered, "Well, I was cast in the TV show *Hollyoaks.*" I thought I was doing very well with one match in particular until she asked where I see myself in five years (I never even know where I'll be the next day). I answered, "Probably a newer version of Minder." I was immediately unmatched.

I started to feel a bit disappointed that my Muslim dating-app experiment wasn't going to plan, especially since I had been so confident at first. In fact I started to feel exactly the same as when I used mainstream dating apps. I had fallen into the same trap of British television producers who think anything Muslim or "BAME" (Black, Asian, and minority ethnic) is completely different from the white norm, when we're essentially all the same. Of course there were different terms being thrown around, and the criteria being used to determine that I wasn't good enough sounded different, but it basically felt the same.

I can't deny the many positives of modern app-based dating as a quick and easy way to find seemingly similar people looking for love (or sometimes just love for one night), but I've found the process incredibly intense and exhausting. The way things are going, it feels like we're heading for a *Black Mirror*-style sci-fi future, where we'll be automatically matched with people we have to marry through an app. But before that happens, I would much rather be brave and try to meet someone in real life. This may seem like an old-fashioned approach, but patience is the key— even if it means a few more years of pretending to laugh at family friends joking about me "being next," and running out of the room whenever my mum brings up the topic of marriage.

RACE & ETHNICITY

JULIA We heard a lot of stereotypes and a lot about how they're untrue.

SHAINA Yeah. I thought it was really interesting to hear from people about how their race or ethnicity was fetishized.

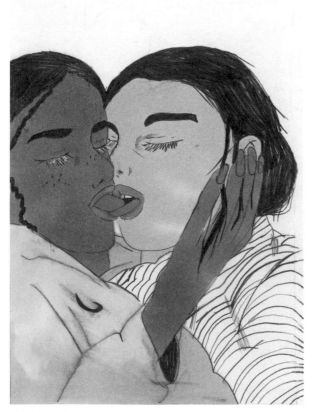

Melek Zertal

I've dated some white women who are into me because I'm Middle Eastern. They have "sand fever." This one woman I dated was into me because it pissed off her family. **Her dad actually called me a "towel head," so I think it was a real turn-on for her.**

Black guys know how to move. It's all about the action. White guys don't know how to move, but they make so much noise: *Ohhhh, yesss. Mmmmmm.* So much noise, but with less action. I try not to laugh when I'm having sex with a white guy.

Everyone thinks Asian men's penises are smaller, but that's not true. Same as everyone else. Some are bigger, some are smaller. Asian men love nasty sex. Dirty things.

Choking is an interesting conversation to have. My girlfriend and I are trying to figure that out. We also have the added element of race—I'm Latina and she's white. I've always been into white girls. I feel like I'm letting down my team, but what can I do? **Anyway, I've noticed that white women love to be choked.** White femmes love a good choke. And now my girlfriend and I are trying to figure out choking stuff. I feel like she's into it because she wants to be submissive in the bedroom because she has all this white guilt, and I think she wants to be dominated because normally she's the dominant one—in the world. Whereas I'm like this immigrant kid in the world. So she has this desire to be physically overtaken. We're very different. She wants to be choked, and I'm like, *I can't even come loudly!*

I used to love nerdy white guys—that's who I lost my virginity to. But then I had a boyfriend who was a dark-skinned African dude, and mostly I've been doing that. It had been years since I was with a white guy, and then a couple of weeks ago I hooked up with one. **I forgot how thin their lips are!**

I go out for drinks regularly with a longtime friend from work. We shoot the shit and vent about work. It doesn't happen that often, but every once in a while we'll get looks from middle-aged white men. **That's when I'm reminded of the fact that my friend is a white female and I'm a black male.** This doesn't happen when I'm out with my white male friends. Once or twice I've noticed a black female bartender give looks when I'm out with a white or Asian female friend or colleague.

I had multiple girlfriends whose parents threatened to stop them from dating me because of my race. I had the most education in the room, but they still treated me like I was 50 Cent—gangbanging—I mean pre-fame, 'hood 50 Cent, not superstar 50 Cent. They would go to the first media generalization, no matter how you presented yourself.

I dated a Jewish woman seriously. Her parents were from Israel. They made it known that they wanted her and her sister to date Hebrew-speaking Jews. One time her parents were away when we had just started dating, and we decided to take a getaway to their place for the weekend. We were out back and she mentioned something about race and her parents—that they wouldn't approve of her dating a black man—and I made us leave right then. Out of principle. If they were not comfortable with her dating a black man, I wasn't comfortable in their home.

That was the beginning of my girlfriend being exposed to race. It took her mom almost a year to even touch me. She would hug her other friends. She would only say *Hi* and *Bye* to me. I was in my mid-twenties. I had dealt with racism my entire life. I had dealt with other girlfriends' parents before. This wasn't new. I always liked them; they were from a different time and place, and very smart. Her dad came around first, while her mom held out. Eventually they realized I wasn't going anywhere. They tried to force their kids, but both kids wound up doing the opposite of what their parents wanted. Her sister married a multiracial woman. To this day, that ex-girlfriend thanks me for being open about it all.

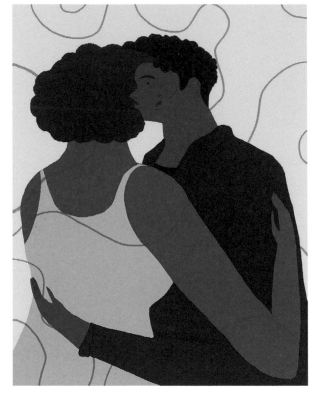

Loveis Wise

I'm a multiracial male. I am lighter-skinned. While I'm definitely black by American standards, I'm far from America's blackest man. I'm also educated. And I do "white" activities, like skating. I wear Vans. I wear short-shorts and bright shirts. I come off as safe and familiar.

In a bar, it's almost a cliché, but there's always a curious white woman. I have to do very little to have an encounter with her.

It happened so often, it became a pattern. I was in the bar to have a good time and drink. **I was never into approaching women. It wasn't my style.** I wouldn't dare put my neck out for rejection. I would just hang out with friends, and sooner or later some white woman would come up to me. Once I realized she was into me, I could turn it on and let down my guard.

It's not like it wasn't the same with other races—it happened with Asians and Indians, too—but white women were the easiest way to sex for me. Black women were attracted to me, but they knew the vibe I was giving off. How I was dressed, they knew I wasn't going to be into them. I got hit on by black women, but I guess it wasn't what I was after. With a white woman, I knew I was going to be in the dominant position.

My sister is black. I grew up around twenty strong black women. I also grew up around race in America. Black women have it the worst out of any other category of how we classify people in this country. I think deep down, I didn't want my sexual deviance to impact black women on top of what they already deal with. I just didn't want to disrespect them in that way. I didn't feel the same with white women—they had all this privilege. It's not like I thought about all of this in the moment. These are all patterns I look back at and wonder about.

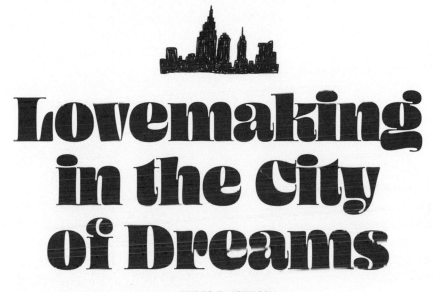

Lovemaking in the City of Dreams

by **MYLES E. JOHNSON**

The idea of living a cliché was living a dream for me. The clichés of a life in New York City were more electric and erotic than life in Georgia. I wanted to work like a New Yorker, think like a New Yorker, and—most importantly to the romantic inside me—I desperately wanted to love like a New Yorker.

The constant search for pleasure can be its own kind of obsession, even if the pleasure is not found. I've found it is possible to be addicted to being insatiable. The constant excitement of never quite having enough or getting it right can easily replace, if you allow it, confronting the emptiness and exhaustion of never locating peace or meaning. Just a constant cycle of *almost*.

This was my problem in New York City. There was plenty of sex, but not a lot of love. It's a city of lights, but it didn't feel like a space to be a light. The concrete jungle hardly produced enough air for me to breathe, let alone thrive. Out of all the lives I led, this was especially disappointing to my love life.

I found myself underneath blue skies and crisp October air—the kind of day that legends like Coltrane and Billie Holiday composed jazz music about. And I was convinced that I was the devil. Not just devilish or prone to demonic thoughts, but *The Devil*. In Park Slope, Brooklyn,

I walked almost four miles attempting to outpace the thought that not only had I forsaken God, but I had done so in many incarnations. This train of thought allowed all the shame and guilt I had ever experienced to resurrect in the front of my mind and guide me into thoughts that I had never allowed to stir my spirit. *Get rid of your bag,* the thought demanded. So I did.

When I thought about what lovemaking would look like in New York City, I imagined a skyline in Manhattan, 'round midnight, with Anita Baker's "Body and Soul" playing as scents of lavender danced between my nostrils, as my lucky lover and I, preferably black and strong, seduced joy from each other with our flesh.

This was my fantasy—and of course the reality was much different.

What I found instead was a motley crew of men willing to make me their plaything, providing nothing more than their dicks to replace my air supply and my ability to communicate. This was A-OK with me, truthfully, because I would rather not show my body. I thought my thighs were too big for a man, or for another man to love. My belly was too big, soft, and round for the serious, sturdy relationship (and lover) I desired. So I allowed myself to be used as a tool to accomplish ejaculation by men denying that they loved other men. They'd explode inside me and I'd let my own imagination erupt with ideas of intimacy that didn't exist.

In honesty, the best sexual experiences I had were alone in my apartment in Crown Heights, door locked, when I was able to divorce my body from my loneliness, usually with the help of porn. This was hardly the big-city romantic fantasy I had in mind.

When I experienced what I now understand was my height of lovemaking in New York City, I was alone, in public, in daylight, surrounded by strangers, feeling far from any type of romance and asking a white woman to help me not die. Like most of my life's experiences, the prophecy that manifested itself and my fantasy didn't look the same, but the lessons were still meaningful and parallel. The quest was still, to quote bell hooks, all about love.

The thought requested that I toss my cell phone, so I did. Following the thoughts caused me brief relief, and I began to be addicted to the short sighs of well-being between mania. The thoughts would subside like a conquered wave until another, more intense thought wave formed and demanded that I surf it. I obliged as the warm sun hit my skin, caressing it—a friend even telling me she was thinking of me as she saw a triple-set of my favorite number (333). I learned even a lovely day couldn't conquer the destiny of a miserable mind.

And then the thoughts avalanched into the biggest demand: to kill myself.

I convinced myself that to fully show my appreciation and remorse to The Divine, I had to go into the woods with nothing and perish. In a moment of mindful clarity that mimicked the autumn day's sky, I witnessed these thoughts compassionately and saw myself as the victim of them, not their creator. And I thought that perhaps before fulfilling this final request for my life, that maybe these philosophical musings were wrong and not to be followed. I stopped walking and I sat outside apartment thirteen. I saw a stranger (who I later learned was named Sarah) entering apartment nine, and I requested her assistance: "I'm having thoughts of killing myself. I've never had thoughts like these before. Can you help me? I'm scared."

Sarah did help. She talked to the police on the phone and assured them I was not armed, then did so again once they arrived by going to the police car before I was even in their sight. Sarah knew that even though I was attempting to overcome tragic thoughts, a black queer man confronting the police could still create a tragedy. This, too, was lovemaking in New York City.

The next couple of days I spent in psychiatric care, negotiating my own mind in the presence of people who appeared to be without their faculties, and wondering what the true difference was, if any. In this space, ableism or any feeling of superiority wouldn't have been just a by-product of bad character or ego, but utterly useless. We were all in the same facility, unable to control the thoughts that would lead us away from our optimal well-being. *Judge not, that ye be not judged* was the recurring thought that I swam.

And there was something freeing about being in group art therapy as a spiritual peer, and understanding that even my intellectual and philosophical muscles could be used against me if I didn't do the work of truly knowing and caring for myself. There is such a thing as being too smart for your own good if you are not good to yourself as you acquire and pursue knowledge. This was me, making love to myself.

It was in a frigid room, with the most uninspiring pale-beige walls, that I sat across from a woman with a ponytail held together by paper she had collected. When I first entered the facility, she was repeating the phrase *kinetic energy* as she paced the hallway. Now she explained how the art she made during group therapy didn't belong to her. She looked at the drawing and then the therapist and said, "This art doesn't even belong to me because it is about my family." She continued, "And it doesn't belong to me now because now it belongs to you." It's always humbling how someone can illuminate a dark corner of your mind with a brief response. I instantly found pleasure in seeing myself as the conduit of a creative message, as opposed to the director or manager of her works. This kind of idea exchange is a form of making love, I thought.

Once released from the psych ward, I bounced between friends' homes. Each friend took their time looking into my eyes and stumbling over words like *nuts* and *crazy* now that I might be one of *those* people. Any time I gazed into the nothingness to clear my mind or expressed the discomfort that anxiety might have delivered to my belly or chest, I was asked if I had taken medication before anything further was discussed.

And even more intimate—I slept in many beds. I was comforted by the unique scents and scenes each friend conjured in their bedroom. During those seven days, I had the courage to know peace only when I lay next to someone who loved me—cried for me—even when I was broken and had buried any promise I had in a seemingly bottomless pit of anxiety and existential doom. They somehow found space in their bed for my spirit, even when my most miserable version of my mind was at the steering wheel.

It's not just about them lying with me, although they did. It's not about them feeding me (literally and spiritually), although they did. It's not about them crying for me, right before they forced me to dance, sing, pray, and dance once again. It's about being enveloped in the energy of people who have decided to love you *until*. To bear witness to your light until your mind has returned from the basement. For seven days I experienced this relentlessly, and I am still climbing. This was the ultimate lovemaking in New York City.

And then I called my mama in Georgia and heard her voice. I was comforted and assured. That was love.

I've consciously practiced celibacy and have learned to see my softness—my belly, my thighs, my personality—as gifts to be offered to the observer of my beauty, not just any seeker of pleasure who scrolls past my photograph. Hating myself and returning to loving myself has introduced the idea that I am not a consolation prize. Again, this was nothing like my fantasy. But the lesson remains that love and true erotic pleasure aren't something to search for, but something to make where you find yourself.

MENTAL HEALTH

SHAINA I get depressed a lot.

JULIA I cry a lot. And I suffer from a lot of anxiety.

SHAINA Oh, I get anxious too. What do you do to stop your anxiety?

JULIA I go outside and hang out with other people and I try to remember that it will go away soon.

SHAINA I'm just the opposite: I feel like I need to be alone and go inside myself. When I'm feeling depressed, it's hard to remember that I don't always feel that way. But eventually I do start to feel a little better, and then little by little I get back into my life.

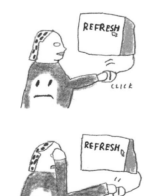

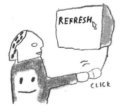

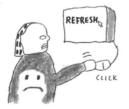

Jon-Michael Frank

If anyone you know needs confidential mental-health support, you can contact the National Helpline at 800.273.TALK (800.273.8255).

My father passed away two years ago. That's been tough for me. But my life is turning around in such a positive way, and I've made such strides. **And the one thing I really learned from him is that real love is a real thing—it can happen.** My parents met and were together for thirty-three years. I do believe that there's someone for everyone.

I managed to get to twenty-six without having sex, but I wouldn't say it was a choice. I was always super-shy. _I've wanted a boyfriend since I was eighteen, but it's never happened._ Being an introvert and having low confidence, it's not been easy. I consider myself an attractive girl and a nice person, but it seems that's not enough, and that's depressing. I want sex, but with my problems and overwhelming lack of confidence, I'm in such a dark place that I don't see it happening. I've decided I'm not going to just "get it over with"; I need to be attracted to them, and things need to be right.

My husband, David, and I lost our son in a tragic car accident a little over a year ago. From the moment we found out, every aspect of our lives has been turned upside down as we try to process this loss. Our son was taken from us along with the future we thought we had with him. We felt as if we had been robbed. Everything became difficult: getting out of bed, eating, breathing, hanging out with friends, going out in public, going to work.

Family members felt for us, but they didn't know how to deal with our pain and were sometimes insensitive. Friendships suffered because who the hell knows how to deal with this kind of thing? In the beginning, we would forget to eat—all day long, no food. By the time we realized we should eat something, it was too late and we just went to bed rather than expend the energy to cook. We struggled with how to move forward with broken hearts, how to navigate a world without our son. It felt like we would go crazy from grief.

When I asked about the nonstop crying, a friend who had lost a kid told me, "As long as you're functioning, it's okay." And eventually—somehow, some way—we began to function: we took walks in the park, we met with friends, we went to the movies.

Sadly, it was all a front. We were all about getting through the day, longing for bedtime so we could end the nightmare of the waking hours. Life was joyless for a while there. The light was gone, and we were walking through a fog; there was a haze over everything. We wanted to retreat from the world, from ourselves, from each other.

About two months after our son died, we tried having sex. I didn't really want to, but I was trying for my husband; he wanted to and needed to feel loved by me. I pretty much cried the entire time. We tried again a few weeks later—same thing. We tried a third time and it was a little better, but still I cried. I didn't feel right doing it; I felt a sense of

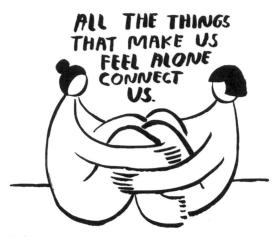

ALL THE THINGS THAT MAKE US FEEL ALONE CONNECT US.

Carissa Potter

guilt for doing something that is supposed to bring so much pleasure. Without discussing it, we just put sex away. I decided I was not going to continue trying to do something I knew I couldn't handle.

Thankfully, my husband respected this nonverbal decision. We have always had a healthy sex life, so it was strange not having sex. I had to learn to put aside the guilt I felt for not having sex with him so that I could take care of myself—to grieve in the way I needed to. **We continue to cuddle and hold hands and touch, see each other naked after a shower, take naps snuggled in on the couch, but there's nothing sexual to it.** It's been about a year with no sex, and we are okay. I am still not ready for it, but I have a feeling something may happen soon.

The other day I was telling David about a friend of mine who was leaving her partner (they'd been having difficulties for a while now and had stopped having sex). He looked up at me from where he was sitting and with a look of torment on his face said, "We aren't having sex either."

"Yeah," I said, "but it's not over; we *will* have sex again."

I went to him and we hugged and I cried.

In the seven years I was with my husband, I never had an orgasm during sex. When our marriage ended, I started dating a man I always had a spark for and the sex was incredible—orgasms left and right. Such fierceness as well as tenderness; we were so in love from early on. He was a tall and beautiful man, had strong yet peaceful hands that knew just how to touch me. There were so many times when we would come at the same moment —it felt magical.

Ten years later he got cancer, and our relationship changed when I became his caregiver. Instead of getting closer and opening up to me, he pulled away and was angry and bitter for having to lie in bed all day. For being in so much pain. For knowing he wasn't ready to leave but being forced to. It wasn't *all* sour: we still said "I love you" countless times a day, still held hands and kissed often, still laughed and joked around and started fun new routines and habits. **I'm ashamed to admit that I started resenting him, and our morphing relationship, a little bit.** I can't pretend I had even an inkling of what he was going through internally, and I'm trying to curb my feelings of guilt at how I felt about him at times.

From his diagnosis on, I gave him only a couple of blow jobs. We no longer had that sexual desire for each other; instead it transformed into a primal need for giving and receiving care.

It hasn't quite been a year since he died, and how I desperately miss his beautiful warm body lying next to me! I miss smelling his delicious skin and feeling his fingers fit perfectly inside me. I miss how he would hold me, how he would pick me up like I weighed nothing, the way he sleepily said my name after an orgasm. I feel like I'll never feel anything like that again, but somehow that's okay. I was lucky enough to feel that for ten years—what an incredible gift I was given.

I've had a diagnosed generalized anxiety disorder (GAD) for seven years now, since I was in high school. My therapist recommended that I learn yoga and progressive muscle relaxation to get rid of stress, but I never really got into those things. On the other hand, I've felt attracted to kink like bondage and submission for some years now, but I never knew how to experience those interests, because— of course—I was afraid, and those interests felt contrary to being afraid most of the time.

I had some experiences with guys who weren't really into this subject; with guys who were into it but not very sensible; and with girls who were afraid to do things like this with me because of my GAD. So in August of this year, I decided to go to a rope-bondage workshop with my best friend in Berlin. **This unusual activity—sharing my sexual interests with a stranger—was weird in my mind, but the teacher was warm and I trusted her.** So I learned how to tie legs and arms. During class I felt unusually relaxed. The teacher told us that many of her customers practice rope bondage for relaxation; it doesn't have to be sexual. That statement opened my eyes! Being tied up could help me cope with my anxiety?

I tried this out with my best friend. From the moment I am tied up, my mind gets calm. It works every time. Rope bondage is an unusual coping strategy, but I also like it in a sexual way.

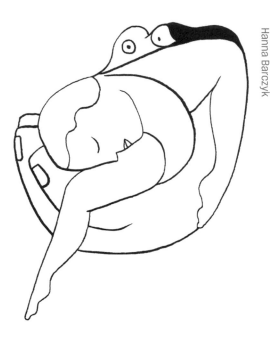

Hanna Barczyk

I've been bulimic for the past nine years. **I've been happy with my body recently, but I still have days when I am unhappy and go back to the habit of throwing up.** My family still doesn't know, because I always doubted how they would react and try to understand; Korean culture doesn't fully recognize the importance of upbringing and mental/physical health.

This was hard for me to grasp when I needed help through the years, but I learned that there's so much other support around me. I've learned to trust my friends more, and to heal through meditation and reading. I now have hopes that I will be able to share with my family sometime in the future.

I suffered from bulimia and anorexia from fifteen years old until I was twenty-four. Only now (I'm thirty-two) have I accepted that it wasn't completely my fault. I had a super-crazy childhood: lived on two continents by the age of ten, had super-young parents who fought and cheated in front of me and my sister. Also, sexual abuse and depression run in my family. It was a terrible illness, and I thought it would kill me. But after several years of therapy and recoveries, I am finally healthy, and I've achieved some incredible things: I'm currently doing a PhD in economics, running research in Africa.

Funny enough, this mental illness became a sort of power, because stressful situations don't really push me away: I've already seen the worst I can get, and I know anything from outside can't get me to that place. Probably that's why I seem so "fearless" to other people. The truth is that I still fear things, but there is nothing—*nothing*—scarier than a mental disease. When I say this to myself, everything seems small.

I was hanging out with family members—drinking wine and celebrating my birthday—and I got really drunk. After that, we went to a bar, I remember taking a shot of something, then I completely blacked out. **I woke up and came to in a stranger's house.** We were in a unique position, having sex—actually anal sex, which I had never done before. I pushed him away a little bit. I didn't even know his name. I wanted to run out of there. He started apologizing, saying, *Please give me your name and number, I'll call you sometime,* but I just wanted to run out of there. I ended up leaving my underwear behind and everything and doing a walk of shame, because it was about eight in the morning and I had to go to work.

It was a really wild night, but it's like it never happened—I never told my friends. I don't remember his face; I didn't want to look at it. I didn't even want to know his name!

I was ashamed of myself for a very long time. It was the kind of night when I think anything could have happened, so I'm glad I'm alive to even say this. It was an eye-opener. That's when I realized I needed to not drink anymore. I needed to slow down and watch myself. And I am sober now.

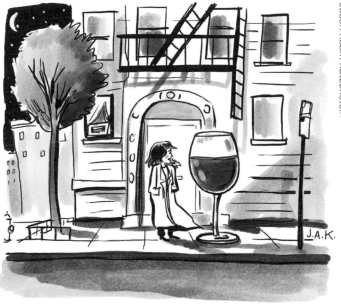

"Would you like to come up and help me call my ex?"

For a long time I needed to be under the influence of alcohol to have sex. Through my twenties, there wasn't a time when I wasn't drunk. They went hand in hand. Because of that dynamic, a lot of my sexual choices and behavior were self-serving. I was always at a bar, I was always drinking. Sex was often how I gained my self-worth. I didn't even know the women. I would remember some of it, but a lot was forgettable.

I wasn't really concerned about the woman, necessarily—though I did always try to use protection—and I feel very fortunate that I didn't get a disease or do anything I regret. Still, I made a lot of horrible choices: it was a lot of waking up in the morning and meeting the woman. We wouldn't have any intimacy until the morning, when the alcohol faded for both of us. It stunted my intimacy and my sexual exploration.

As I get older—I'm in my thirties now—I'm beginning to experience more intimacy. Today I'm sober, and it's a lot different for me. As I feel more comfortable with who I am, I'm able to open up more. It's wonderful. It's so much better.

BODY

10 THINGS TO DO WHEN YOU'RE HORNY & LONELY

by Fareeha Khan

drawings by Julia Rothman

1. Read a book about attachment theory, identify heavily with the idea of the "anxiously attached" lover stuck in a cycle of chasing after the "avoidant" lover. Realize this is why you've felt constantly heartbroken for years.

2. Really let that sink in. I mean, really, dude. That heartbreak sucks absolute ass. Decide you need to take a break from dating to clear your mind and assess these patterns of behavior you've been engaged in for far too long.

3. Relish in quality "you" time — sleep in, read books, get into astrology, watch whatever the hell you want on TV in your underwear.

4. Months into your new liberating lifestyle, suddenly register that although now you do love being alone, you're actually quite horny and quite lonely. Learn the definition of "incel." Realize you gotta get back out there.

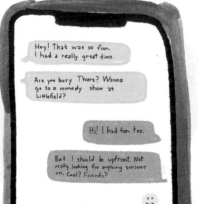

5.

Go on a date with a sweet guy who seems really interested in you. Take things slow. You're different now. Let yourself relax and realize you like him. He can't be avoidant— he's present and cool and takes you on real dates. You're breaking your attachment pattern! Wait to hook up until date three. Who are you? A hero? DAMN. That's awesome. You're killing it.

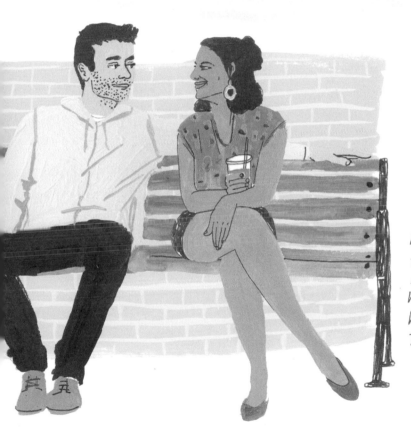

6. He texts you the next day to say he doesn't want anything serious. Notice that despite all the work you've done on yourself, that rejection still hurts. Feel a bit discouraged that you didn't break the cycle ... yet. Feel foolish... Let it sting.

Hey! That was so fun. I had a really great time.

Are you busy Thurs? Wanna go to a comedy show at Littlefield?

Hi! I had fun too.

But I should be upfront. Not really looking for anything serious rn. Cool? Friends?

7. Go back to your incel lifestyle. You're alone a lot, but working through shit. You're facing your fears. You're not a coward.

8. Buy a vibrator. A really good one. You deserve it! Get back into appreciating the glory of free porn on the internet.

9. Go to therapy. Read books. Chase your dreams. Hang out with friends. Go hiking. Have soul-baring conversations with strangers. Believe you can be a better person. Read that Cheryl Strayed book and let her wisdom hit you— "These things are your becoming." Realize that you do get horny and you do get lonely, but that doesn't mean you should settle for anyone unless they realize how incredible you are and you feel the same about them. Go on dates again. Realize the best people are the ones who accept you as you are and are willing to work with you. Cherish this.

10. Love yourself and your people. Life without love sucks absolute ass.

BEING INTERSEX

RIVER GALLO

My name is River Gallo and I am a filmmaker, an actor, a writer, and an intersex advocate. I am from New Jersey originally and live in LA now.

My parents came from El Salvador in 1980—they were escaping the civil war that was happening there. They came illegally. They piled onto an empty gasoline tank with a bunch of other people and then swam across the Rio Grande. When they arrived, they moved from farm to farm in Texas and then eventually got on a bus and went to New York. They lived in New York for a while, and then they ended up moving to New Jersey, having kids, and opening up a Salvadoran restaurant.

I remember distinctly this one time when I was young, my dad, my sister, and I were walking by a car with a Salvadoran flag in it. And my dad said to me and my sister, "We can't do that because then people will know who we are. We can't represent our Salvadoran nationality in America—it's not safe." My parents wanted us to assimilate—they wanted me and my siblings to fit in and not get deported. They wanted us to go to college and do all of these things that white people could do that my parents couldn't do. So even though I grew up in their restaurant and with Salvadoran traditions, there was also a sense of hiding it.

And there were other hidden things about my identity. When I was twelve years old, I went for a doctor's appointment—for allergies or a cold—something unrelated to my genitals. And I remember the doctor saying to my mom, "When do you plan on telling him?" And my mom was like, "Oh, soon." And I was like, *What the fuck are you guys talking about?* It felt like there was this big secret that I didn't know about.

A few weeks later we had another appointment, and it was then that they told me I'd been born without testicles and would need to start doing hormone-replacement therapy. They put me on testosterone. A few years later, when I was sixteen, I had plastic surgery to put prosthetic testicles in my scrotum. It all became something that I was self-conscious of. It was a secret—something I didn't speak to anybody about. I talked to doctors about it when I had appointments, but otherwise I didn't speak about it.

The word *intersex* was never spoken to me until I was twenty-six or twenty-seven. I was writing my thesis film, *Ponyboi*, for grad school, and I thought to myself, *Maybe there's some new research on my condition.* I wanted to incorporate that personal aspect of myself into the script, so I looked online. That's when I stumbled upon this Buzzfeed video with a bunch of intersex advocates—Hanne Gaby Odiele and Pidgeon Pagonis. They were all explaining what *intersex* means and how there's an intersex community and how the UN has declared extreme human-rights violations on these surgeries that doctors say are necessary but are really just cosmetic. These surgeries are done simply so intersex people can fit into the binary of what a typical male or female should look like. So I saw this online and I was like, *Oh my god—I'm intersex!* That's when I realized the surgery I had was not consensual—I never asked for it. It was done to me because they said that's what I needed in order to be a man, but it wasn't consensual.

Just to back up a bit: at eighteen I had come out as gay, then soon after that I identified as queer, and then as nonbinary. So to have a surgery that made me look *more* binary really rattled me. It made me not trust the medical world. It felt like these doctors were complicit in erasing my intersex identity, like they had medicalized it as opposed to giving it a human form. They hadn't been up-front about it at all; they didn't tell me that a lot of what they were claiming was necessary was actually just cosmetic. That had lasting psychological effects on me. So ten years after my surgery, when I found out about being intersex that night when I was doing research for my film, I became an intersex advocate.

When I was younger, before I found out, I didn't know I was any different. I thought my body was my body. But once I found out, I felt disillusioned and betrayed. I felt like the people I trusted most in the world—my parents and doctors—had lied to me my whole life, because they did. They had held back a truth about me and my body. We feed children all this bullshit—the Tooth Fairy, Santa Claus—treating them like they're dumb, but children have more intelligence than we give them credit for. We owe it to children to show them integrity, and to be honest about what we know about them and their bodies.

So when *Ponyboi* happened, there was all this momentum behind it because here I was, this filmmaker who had discovered they were intersex while making a film. Through this whole discovery, I started becoming friends with all of these intersex advocates around the world, and I became a youth advocate with Interact, which is a nonprofit advocacy group for intersex people. It was a great feeling to be connecting like that. For the first time I had people to talk with about the one thing that I had never had a space for. There were people who understood me, who had similar trauma and scars and wounds. For so long we were made to seem like "the other," and we had to keep things secret. But now we don't.

I only recently told my dad what *intersex* is, and that I'm an intersex advocate. I told my mom last year and she's been such an ally to me and so supportive. At first it took a lot of work to dismantle the notions of gender binary in my mom. I'd come home with my hair and nails done and she'd be like, "Why are you doing that?" And I was like, "Listen, Mom, you have to get on board because this is how I choose to express myself." And she got on board. When my movie premiered at Tribeca, I was staying with her in New Jersey, and my mom curled my hair for the premiere. She dropped me off at the nail salon to get my nails done. It was beautiful! And then she came with me to the screening. That was the first time my mom had seen my film, and I had underestimated how hard it would be to show it to her. But she loved it, and she said to me, "Wow—you're such a good actor." I feel like I am on my way to living out my dreams as an artist and, for me, I've discovered that tapping into this vulnerable side of myself is what has helped me to achieve that dream.

When I came out as nonbinary and intersex, I said to myself, *You know what? I'm gonna be very open about these things in terms of dating.* So I was very open about it and on the dating apps I was getting so much attention— specifically from guys who are into feminine or trans-identifying people. It became this very interesting journey of dating and hooking up with guys who are not comfortable with their sexuality, who consider themselves straight and have all these regulations of how they want their partners to look: they want their partners to be completely shaven and made-up. They need all of this in order to uphold these fragile concepts of their masculinity. It's pretty toxic.

All of that is to say, I got a lot of dick pics!

After dating like this for some time, I came to terms with the fact that I couldn't be on dating apps anymore. I couldn't expose myself to this anymore. When I was actively dating, I was explaining intersex to people all the time. And as an oftentimes feminine-presenting nonbinary person, I am often mistaken by people as trans. Like they can understand what *trans* is, but they couldn't understand *intersex* and because they couldn't categorize me as something they understood, it made them nervous. I find that dating apps make me feel like I am reduced to some two-dimensional form. So for my own sanity, I decided to stop being on them. But I'm very interested in dating, and I'm still figuring out how. My priority now, though, is finding intimate connections with people, despite how terribly horny I am!

SEXUAL IDENTITY, ORIENTATION & EXPLORATION

SHAINA I experimented a lot and eventually wound up married to a guy.

JULIA I wish I'd experimented more.

SHAINA There's still time!

I was thinking today, *Maybe I'm not gay.* **I've had really bad experiences with men.** But then I remembered the first time I kissed a woman and I was like, *Oh yeah—that was crazy.*

I identified as a lesbian/stud/butch when I was fifteen years old, then started taking testosterone at twenty-two and started identifying as a trans male. **It was interesting becoming a man after having so many traumatic relationships with men.**

At first when I became a lesbian, I was conditioning myself to be like a man. And then I was like, *Oh, no—I have to unlearn all of this toxic masculine shit.* **I had to unlearn being shitty to women.**

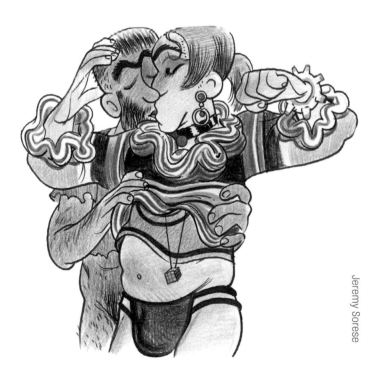

Jeremy Sorese

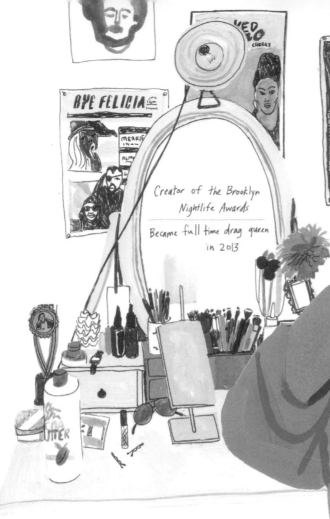

Merrie Cherry →

I moved to New York nine years ago. I was working as a database administrator and doing coat check at the Metropolitan Bar at night. One night I put on some lipstick, a little blush, and a crazy wig. Some drunk woman came up to me and was like, 'You're beautiful,' and she gave me a $20 bill. These explosions went off in my head! So the next night, I put a little more on and people were just tipping me for being in the look.

Julia Rothman

I am a sex-positive asexual. People always say that's contradictory, but I am comfortable with my orientation.

It took me a long time to come to this conclusion. There were lots of second thoughts, confused partners, and self-hate.

I didn't have my first kiss until I was seventeen. I've had one, maybe two crushes my entire life. I had sex for the first time when I was twenty-one. I thought there was something wrong with me, because everybody else was dating and having sex in high school and college. When I learned what asexuality was, everything started making sense—until I started dating.

I came out as ace (asexual) to my first boyfriend after I had a panic attack when he tried to kiss me. I was twenty-one. I cried to my friends on the phone because he said he couldn't be with someone who was ace, and I hated myself for not having sexual feelings toward him. I wanted to change so badly, and cried myself to sleep. The next day he decided to end it.

I ended up begging him to come back and telling him I would have sex with him, but we just needed to move at my own pace. Six months into our relationship we finally had sex, and while I have no regrets, I felt nothing.

I wasn't repulsed, just indifferent. I loved him romantically, so I kept having sex to make him happy, but it didn't make *me* happy. Sex felt like almost nothing—simply a constant pressure that I could entertain for a few minutes before I got bored. I would let him get on top, and it was over when he was finished. I knew it wasn't "normal" to

feel nothing, so I faked everything. I was so insecure I never fully opened myself up to him.

After my first relationship ended, I started casually dating on Tinder, trying to understand what sex meant to me. I told myself to try sleeping with different and new people, and maybe I'd start liking it more. I went on a spree of swipes and a few one-night stands, but I couldn't find that spark. Trying to reach an orgasm felt like a chore every time.

I eventually began a friends-with-benefits relationship, which turned into the most confusing relationship I've been in—but also the most rewarding. My partner never pressured me to orgasm or do things I didn't want to do. He made me feel comfortable in my own body and never acted disappointed when I couldn't come. We talked openly about my asexuality and how I was trying to work through some confusion. He was completely open and made me feel valid. Our ambiguous, open/poly "situationship" was the first relationship that made me feel valid. The stigma surrounding sex had been lifted.

I still have a hard time articulating what sex means to me. It's not a physical thing, but a mental thing. I don't find bodies or people sexually attractive, I don't fantasize about it, and I don't receive pleasure from it.

People ask me why I still have sex if I don't experience that attraction. I am still working on that answer, but sometimes it's the feeling of completely lacking insecurities and having total trust in someone. Sometimes simply pleasing my partner makes me feel sexy and confident. Whatever the reason, I'm happy and comfortable in my sexuality as a sex-positive asexual.

Nearing the end of winter break in 2016, I was a bored nineteen-year-old stuck in suburban Texas. **Back at my liberal arts college hundreds of miles away, I was openly queer and existed in queer communities that supported and validated me.** But at home, I had hardly even thought about coming out. I knew my parents would be accepting, kind—enthusiastic, even—but I had always been private with my family (about love and relationships especially), and as my parents were going through a divorce, my queerness wasn't a can of worms I wanted to open.

I was the oldest. My little sister often cried about her problems, but I felt like I needed to keep it together and keep any issues to myself. Then on a sunny Tuesday in late January, my fourteen-year-old sister refused to let me go to the movies with her. I couldn't believe it. Here I was, home from college, and she didn't even want to spend time with me! I was trying to put effort into our relationship, but she was not reciprocating. I stormed into my room like the mature college kid I was, angry, until

she came into my room in tears a few minutes later. Sitting on my bed, the winter sun pouring into my childhood room, she said through sobs that she had wanted to see a gay movie and didn't want me to judge her for it. She said she was gay, but that she was afraid I would see her differently, or that I wouldn't love her in the same way.

These were words I understood so much more than she knew—and they were breaking my heart. All at once I felt a rush of emotions, one of them being a wave of gut-wrenching guilt. I had always thought that keeping things to myself—problems, experiences, my queer identity—was the humble, considerate, low-maintenance thing to do. But as my little sister came out to me, her gay big sister, I realized that isn't always the case. Our relationship as sisters had felt disconnected for a while—we were in different places, into different things—and now more than ever I mourned all the hours and days and years of connecting over our shared queer identity we had missed because I had been too shy (or too proud, or too scared,

or too busy) to tell her that I was gay. And then a wash of joy came over me as I realized all the time we had ahead of us to build this connection, to giggle about crushes on girls, to know that despite our differences, this is an identity we share.

Years have passed since my little sister's brave words that winter afternoon, and I'm still working on being open with myself and the people I love. It seems like a simple lesson, but now I know that while silence can be more comfortable, it's when we speak that we reach the people around us, and it's through that courage that we find love and connection

Recently, I told this story to a friend, and she reminded me that while being open is brave and important for yourself and others, it's also okay if you aren't ready to be. So I don't feel guilty anymore about not coming out to my little sister sooner; I just wasn't ready—and that's okay. Now, though, I remind myself to not be so quiet. Sometimes talking about yourself is exactly what someone around you might need to hear.

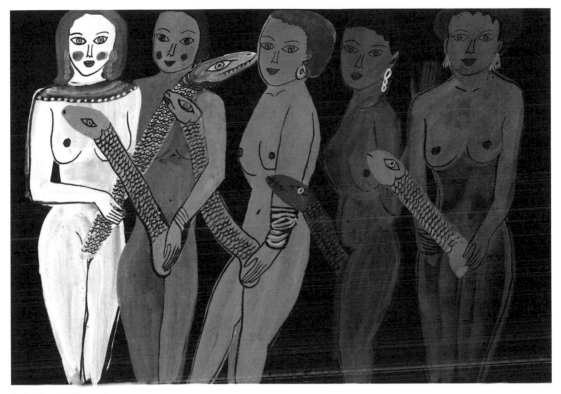

Arrington de Dionyso

E was, and is, the first woman I've ever fallen for. **I've always been attracted to women, I think, but never pursued it because I figured that attraction was more of an appreciation.** She'd had crushes on women before, but never knew how to name it. We stumbled into each other, emotionally and physically. It took us months of touching and kissing to admit to each other, *Are we having sex?*

Neither one of us had ever been with a woman before. We'd never really watched porn. I knew I'd had sex with my boyfriend, because when you stick a penis in a vagina, *Bam!* Sex! And when I was "too tired" with (of?) him and we went to bed after a hand job or light fingering, we didn't *actually* have sex, right? So how do you define it when there is no penis in play? E and I had no idea. It felt weird and bad and silly and good and scary and awkward that I couldn't define sex with her. I love books and devoured all the queer lit I could, looking for answers (a heartfelt thank-you to *Fun Home* and *Blue Is the Warmest Color*). Finally I decided this: if we are both orgasming, we are having sex.

Five years have gone by, and no one has ever confirmed or denied this for us. If she's not in the mood but I am, and she makes me come, did we have sex? You can have sex with yourself, you can have sex with someone(s) else, but in the previous situation, is she having sex with me if only one person comes? Am I having sex with her?

When I think about these things it makes my head spin, but it also makes me laugh. Will I ever know the answers to my specific queer sex questions? We're happy, and I think that's enough for now.

The first time I remember orgasming, I was eleven years old and it was while thinking of a woman. My hometown is small, conservative, and located right in the middle of the Bible Belt. When I was growing up, I didn't see out-and-proud queer people. The thought of being queer terrified me.

Throughout high school I tried to date boys, and tried hard to get my first kiss so I could prove to myself that I wasn't gay. The kiss didn't happen until my freshman year of college, and the only thing noteworthy about it was the location: on a golf course at 1 a.m. Nevertheless I continued dating men, and when I was nineteen I had sex for the first time, with a guy I met at a party. Afterward he told me, "I wanted to do that so badly that if you hadn't let me, I would have raped you." Exactly one week later, his roommate raped me.

In the year that followed, I decided *Fuck it* and had regular one-night stands with guys, none of which were enjoyable; I never orgasmed. Eventually I stopped having sex altogether and went on masturbating alone while fantasizing about women.

Then I met my ex-boyfriend, who I ended up dating for three years. We waited a full year to have sex with each other, and it was the first time I had an orgasm while having sex with someone other than myself. It was a time filled with love and tenderness. Toward the end of our relationship, our sex life became boring to me—and probably to him too. We ended up talking about our fantasies and he said he was turned on by two women having sex with each other. I agreed it was hot—but didn't disclose that I had thought so since I was eleven! It was the first time I had come close to coming out to anyone. Eventually I couldn't have an orgasm with him unless I was imagining myself having sex with a woman.

After moving to the East Coast and starting grad school, I began app dating and having regular one-night stands with men again. But as was the case in undergrad, I was not orgasming or enjoying myself. One day I tried switching my preferences to *Everyone*. I swiped right on one femme-presenting

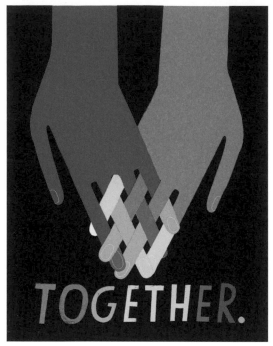

Lisa Congdon

TOGETHER.

person, panicked, then immediately switched back to men only.

Through therapy, I've been able to get to the point where if I'm on an app for dating, I can have my preferences set to only *Women* without feeling that sense of fear and panic. **I told my friends and my mom that I might start dating women, but I still haven't. Due to my lack of experience, I often don't feel queer enough to say I'm queer, and I'm still learning what being queer can mean.**

After having mostly terrible sex with men, and after being assaulted by a man, I want my first time having sex with a woman to be special. But the fear of *What if it isn't any different?* has kept me from making any moves. So I haven't had sex in seven months, but that feels safest for now. I'm grateful to have queer friends who make me feel loved and like I belong. I'm grateful to see out-and-proud queer couples regularly in the city where I now live. This is already far more than my eleven-year-old self could have ever imagined.

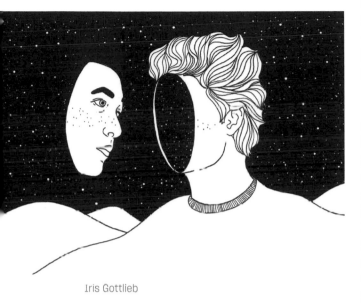

Iris Gottlieb

When I was really young, I fantasized about both boys and girls, but when I got older it was all about the boys. When I went to college at first I was like, *I can't have sex.* I just dry-humped the boys and I was like, *I like this!* I then had sex with a girl; I ate her out—and I was good at it!—but I wasn't that into it. It was hot in the moment, but in the end I was like, *I don't want to kiss a girl's kooka.*

I guess I'm fluid, but I really like dudes more.

I came out to everyone when I was twenty-two. I fought it for a long time. I knew it forever. **I knew I was attracted to boys before I knew what being gay was.** Maybe for a while I thought I was attracted to girls, but mostly I just forced myself. It wasn't real. I had sex with two girls in my life—it was not for me. The first time I had sex with a guy was terrifying. I was twenty-one. It was a Tinder boy. It meant I was finally admitting to myself that I was gay. It was about me accepting that.

I came out when I was eighteen. I didn't kiss a lot of guys—I had sex only once before college—but I was leaning hard into being hetero. **Then I went to college and took this business-law class, where I met my first lesbian.** She had been hooking up with women since she was like twelve, and on the first day of class she sat next to me and said, "You're a lesbian."

And I was like, "No I'm not."

She just worked on me for, like, three months, and eventually she turned me—like a vampire. By May of my first year in college, I was out and had a girlfriend. I think she saw my masculine center—the energy in me. I was always very masculine and a tomboy, but I didn't really have the language to know what I was. I'm not saying that everyone who's like that is queer, but I was, and I just didn't realize it until she came along. I really had no prototype for this when she told me I was a lesbian. It was right when *The L Word* had come out on Netflix, so I binged it, and I was like, *Yep—totally.*

Gay New York is like Tupperware: You can always find a bottom, but you can never find a top.

There are a lot of theories why there are so many bottoms in this town. The most common is that people work long hours at demanding jobs, so they want to be dominated. Thrusting is a lot of work. Tops are in short supply in New York. If you are a top, you are like a Greek god.

I used to flirt with girls when I was a little girl. I was, like, seven and would see these twenty-year-olds, or my teachers, and I was like, *Oh, hell yeah—that's hot!* **But I didn't know what to do with those feelings, so I just acted straight.** I put on capri pants, found a bra that wasn't a sports bra, and found a guy who would kiss me. But when I got older I was like, *Oh, wait a minute—I'm gay!*

I knew I was gay in fifth grade—maybe eleven or ten—when I started catching feelings for one of my friends.

I was a week away from my nineteenth birthday and taking the weekend off school to visit NYC with my mother. Given our not-so-great relationship (she was not super-accepting of my sexuality when I came out as gay, and I hadn't told my parents I was nonbinary), I got my own hotel room next to hers instead of sharing. I go to a small school and had been in a very small community before college, so I hadn't had much experience with girls and was too nervous to use Tinder at school. So because I was in NYC for the weekend, I decided to take advantage of the situation and swipe through Tinder. *Why not? Maybe it would even go somewhere and I'd finally get some.*

Saturday night after dinner my mom went right to sleep in the room next to me while I set up an embarrassingly clichéd profile and started swiping. After a while the swiping became mindless, matching with people every so often and sending the same *Hey, how's it going?* message every time. Then a trans guy from Tisch (NYU's art school) messaged back and we started talking. He said he would have invited me over if his roommates weren't there, so I invited him over instead. I had never been attracted to a guy, but he was kind of cute and seemed into

me (which is always a plus), so I brought him up to my room. We started making out, one thing led to another, and I lost my virginity to him, with my mother in the next room none the wiser.

Honestly, I'm surprised she didn't wake up: I was *not* quiet when his tongue touched my clit, and neither was he when the roles were reversed. We fucked for a while and then he left for a movie night with his roommates—a prosaic end to a certifiable yet successful one-night stand.

If I could go back and change it, would I?

No, probably not.

I had fun and felt good, and virginity is just a social construct that doesn't mean much to me anyway. What is *virginity* for me (a gay, nonbinary, intersex person) anyhow—my first orgasm? Because I had gotten myself there years before. Penetration? Not my thing. Sex with someone I love? Haven't gotten there yet. And why did I fuck a guy for my first time and not a girl? Do I like guys now, too? Probably not— I don't think I'd ever fuck a cis dude—but maybe sexuality is more fluid than we think. **Let's just leave it as a fun night in NYC with orgasms and pussy galore, all while sharing a wall with my homophobic mom.** What. A. Story.

I'm bisexual or gender fluid. **I think love is love.** I've fallen in love with men, women, someone transitioning from male to female. I'm 50 percent masculine and 50 percent feminine. I always knew I was bisexual, but I didn't explore it until I was in college.

When it comes to women's bodies, they are ten times more supple and fun to explore. Men are harder and more sculpted. It's a different terrain. When I'm with women I'm more graceful and slow, and when I'm with men I'm more rough.

From the time I was a teenager to age thirty-three, I thought of sex from a scarcity mentality. My dad was emotionally abusive, and I've lived in a fat body most of my life. **My dad's treatment of women, mixed with the world's treatment of fat people, helped me form the opinion that I would never be worth loving—that I'd better take any crumb resembling love I could get.** I lost my virginity to a guy I met online because I wanted to get it over with. After that, I became part of a lot of what I called "half relationships": friends with benefits…situations where I was the other woman.

I was bi but didn't have much experience with women, so I started hooking up with a lot of women who weren't out except on the internet. I believed then that it added up to feeling loved, but it was like adding a bunch of negative numbers and expecting to come up with a positive: it never worked, and it just left me craving real intimacy and love.

Eventually I started posting ads on Craigslist and having a bunch of anonymous sex. I made sure to post pictures of my body so I could be certain that anyone responding knew what they were getting into. There were lots of times where I'd have somebody over to my apartment and fuck them even if I thought they were gross; that seemed less scary than saying no. I also met people from

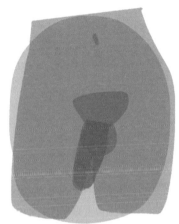

Tio Cuchillos

a porn website that had a social feature—almost like Facebook. I was fetishized a lot for being fat. I hated it. I ended up getting herpes, which felt like a world-ending event at the time but hasn't affected my life in any real way. In total I've had something like sixty partners.

At thirty-three, I realized I didn't want to feel like my sex life was a big secret. I wanted to know what it might be like to be loved in a real way—to start with getting to know somebody instead of starting out with sex. I went to a 12-step program for intimacy stuff, but what helped the most was group therapy with other women, where we learned to practice saying our true feelings. Asking for what we wanted.

Now I'm thirty-seven. I haven't really had sex in four years, with the exception of two times with a partner I've known for years. I don't want to be celibate forever. But things have gotten even more complicated—I now identify as a trans guy. I want somebody to learn my body and what feels affirming alongside me. I haven't undergone a medical transition. That old fear I have about being unlovable comes up a lot. I have destructive thoughts and wonder who could love a trans, fat, herpes-ridden person like me? Then I remind myself of how deeply I believe that we are all inherently lovable, and I let go of the fear as much as I can. But it's hard.

I was outed at, like, twelve.
I had this separate Instagram
account to explore and see if
I'm, like, interested in men.
Someone found the account
and spread it all over school.
So people knew I was at
least some percentage gay
at a very early age. And
to my surprise, everyone was
like, Yeah, cool.

I come from Venezuela; it's a
very macho culture, but they
were accepting of it. It was
weird because I didn't want
to be out, but I was. And
all I received was love.

I had my first gay-sex experience at sixty-seven years old.

This is a true story. I grew up with a very repressed sexuality. I did not date in high school and barely dated in college. I had kissed only one girl. I always wondered if I was gay, but I didn't have a conscious attraction or desire for men. I realize from the vantage point of seventy years that the Catholic seminary was the perfect place to run away from my sexuality and fears about intimacy. But, as has been the case for countless others, things caught up with me, and I left after my first year of graduate school.

In school I met a woman who was eleven years older than me. We fell in love—and we still love each other dearly to this day—but our sex life began to die after the first fifteen years or so of marriage. I always blamed myself. And I learned after I came out that she always blamed *herself*. But neither of us knew how to talk about it.

I met a guy in church. I was instantly attracted to him, which freaked me out completely. He liked me, and we developed a friendship that went on for five years. I constantly suppressed the attraction over those years, but he invaded my fantasy life in a big way, and the few times I masturbated it was to those mental images of him.

We were slated to go to a church convention, and I found myself scheming ways to spend some time with him. I ended up inviting him to share a double-double hotel room, and the way he said yes told me he was onto my schemes.

We arrived at the hotel the day of the convention, dropped our bags, and headed over to the conference center. At the end of the first day's business, we took off and had dinner at Red Lobster. We were both flirting—you could cut the sexual tension with a knife. After dinner we drove back to the hotel, and we both stripped down to our skivvies without saying anything. Finally he asked, "Now what?" I opened my arms; we embraced and kissed. It was like lightning bolts for me. I distinctly remember underwear flying through the air, tongues, hands, hearts pounding, groping, and more kissing. We ended up giving each other blow jobs. He was incredibly gentle. I was like a sixteen-year-old!

After God knows how long, we drifted off to sleep in each other's arms. At some point I woke up laughing, and he asked, "Are you okay?"

Through my giggling I managed to say, "So that is what I am!"

He replied, "I always knew it."

We talked for a long time, shared stories, asked and answered questions, kissing, before drifting off to sleep again.

The next morning I had an amazing revelation: that night with him was the first time in my living memory when sex was free of anxiety. I felt this incredible freedom, this feeling of rightness.

It is no exaggeration to say that my life changed completely in that period of time, culminating in that hotel room. I cherish that memory, and I cling to my newfound identity as a gay man who struggled for decades to emerge from a self-imposed cocoon of repression and suppression. I lost him to COPD in February of 2018, but he certainly lives on in my heart.

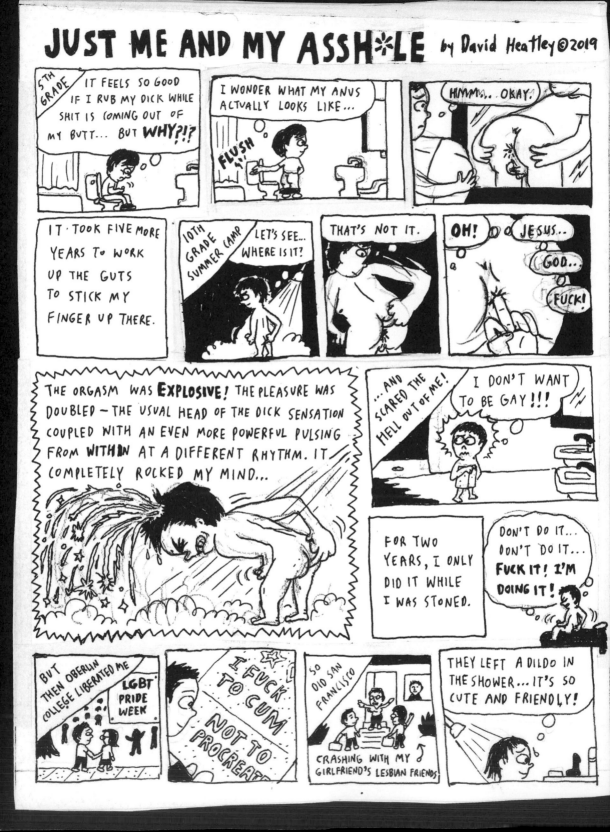

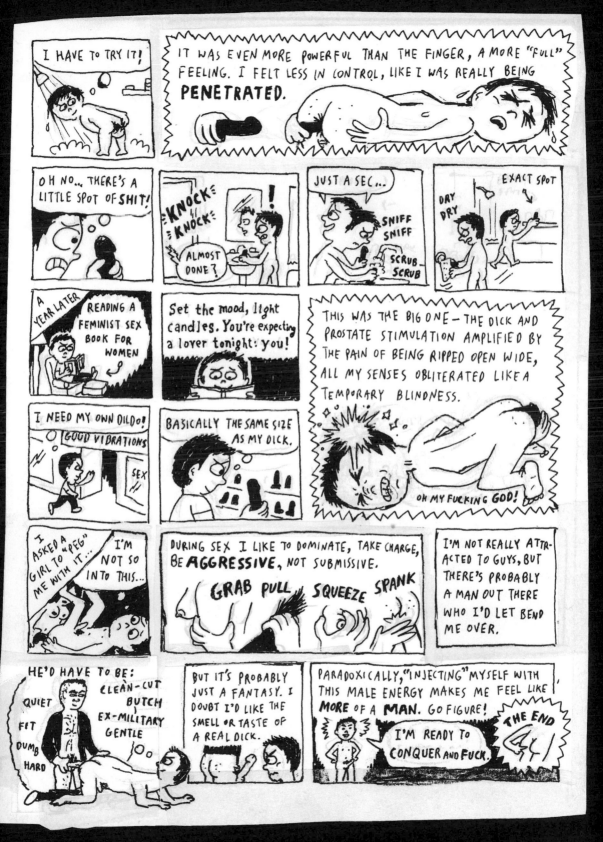

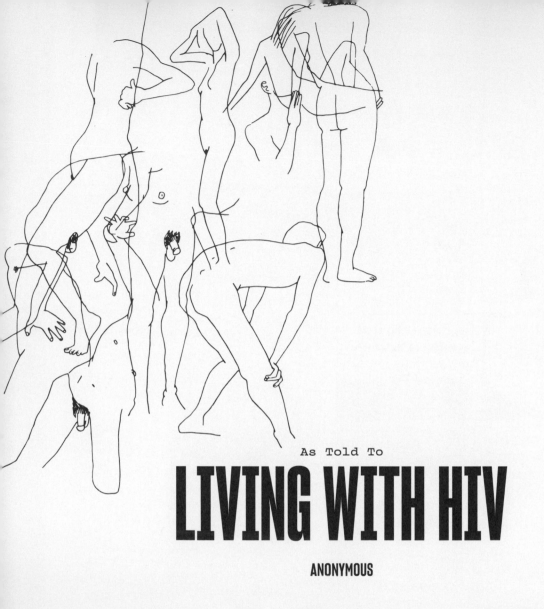

As Told To

LIVING WITH HIV

ANONYMOUS

From my earliest memories, I knew I was gay. I didn't know what it was, but I knew I liked boys and not girls. I'm from a black, Southern, conservative family; lower middle class, private school, music lessons, braces—all that crap. My mother is uber-religious. I knew it wasn't safe or cool to be gay in my family, in that house.

At school I think about 10 percent of the kids were black, and I was in the closet. I was musically gifted, so I played a couple of instruments and became an organist at the church when I was fifteen. After high school I got a music scholarship to university, and that's where I came out. This was in 1982.

Washington, DC, was 70 percent black and incredible, because it was a thriving city with several different classes of black folks. I'd never seen a black judge or a black lawyer. As a black man, I could suddenly do anything. It was very liberating sexually, because I was a gay man in a big city with lots of gay culture, lots of gay clubs, lots of gay bars. And it was great to be gay, to see other beautiful, handsome guys. I went to bars, met guys, slept with them, whatever. Drugs, booze, cigarettes—all that stuff. I came out, I was young, I was beautiful. I had lots of sex.

Around the same time, AIDS hit the city. People would get sick, then they'd be dead in literally two weeks. It was scary. I was nineteen years old, and I knew people who had died.

I was a military dependent, so I was able to go to the military hospital. I knew I kind of had risky sexual behavior, so I'd go every two months to check for STDs. This was pre-condoms; the message *Condoms equal safe sex* hadn't come out yet. Back then we knew you got the disease from having sex, but nobody knew anything else. There was no medication. They started using this new test to see if you had the antibody for HIV, and I had it. So now I'm twenty years old, with a head full of Jesus and mommy guilt and church guilt. So what do I do? I decided I'm just going to party like a rock star, and if I live to see twenty-one that'll be okay.

But I didn't die. I finished university, and in 1986 I moved to New York. My dream was to become a recording engineer. I started going to the Institute of Audio Research in the West Village. I knew I had this disease, but I didn't know the language to express it to people, so I shut down sexually. I started drinking, and drinking, and drinking. And I started doing drugs. It was the eighties, it was New York. There were fabulous clubs like Paradise Garage, so I basically went out clubbing every night. The music was great, the scene was great. It was integrated, it was inclusive. A group of us—straight, gay, boys, girls—would party and just go dancing. I dropped out of school because I didn't like the program, so I got a job working for the city and just partied.

Eventually I got this wonderful boyfriend, and I told him my status; he was okay with it. We weren't really doing safe sex, but looking back we didn't have sex that often. It was much more about intimacy and companionship, and it wasn't very sexual. I was still very sexually shut down. I had really low self-esteem and a lot of self-hatred—because I was gay, because I was HIV-positive, and because I was carrying around this secret I was ashamed of.

I had moved to New York to do music, so I broke up with the boyfriend, got my own place, and bought a keyboard. Music became my salvation. I started meeting DJs and producers and learning how to make dance music—and music saved me. I had some ideas about producing music, and I lost myself in those. Then in '89 I moved into a house in Brooklyn with all musicians. I was starting to hone my musical craft, but my addiction went crazy. I was out in an Italian neighborhood and really isolated. I bottomed out in that apartment. I'd met this straight guy who had just gotten out of jail and needed a place to live, so I moved him in. I came home from work one night and my apartment was totally empty. That was the catalyst to me getting clean. There was a singer I knew who was sober—I called him and he sent me to rehab.

But then, after I'd been sober for a year, I got very sick. I'm five foot ten, but I dropped to about 110 pounds. I looked like death. I couldn't keep anything in my system. No energy, no appetite. This friend of mine told me about a clinic near East Broadway where you could go and get acupuncture. Two Chinese doctors there—women—nursed me back to health. I was on disability because I couldn't do anything, so I went and got acupuncture and Chinese herbs and massages, and I took all these supplements. I learned how to take care of myself—physically, mentally, spiritually. I learned proper nutrition. I went to therapy to deal with my fucked-up head. Eventually I got strong enough to take the cocktail [of antiretroviral drugs].

I tell people that HIV was one of the greatest things to ever happen to me. I know that sounds weird, but it made me grow up. You can be a gay man and never grow up—live in a world of sex and drugs your whole life, and never have to face anything. HIV gave me the gift of having to look at myself. I had to get sober. Had to go to therapy. Had to sort out my low self-esteem. Had to repair the anger and hurt I had with my folks. It saved my life.

I think a sad thing that I see, being a gay man at fifty-five, is there's two generations after me who don't know anything about this. They don't know what it's like to have all your friends die. They don't know the pain of caring for someone who is sick, watching them wither. I saw my blond model friend go from 220 to 119 and resembling a starving kid in three months. A lot of people don't have that reference. These days they're on PrEP [pre-exposure prophylaxis] and don't even have to use condoms. We went through purgatory—the ones who are still left, that is.

Throughout the years, I've had HIV-positive guys write me for advice. I tell them, "Take the time to get to know the disease—what it does, what the treatments are. It's not a death sentence but a wake-up call, and it can be a wonderful opportunity to grow. You don't usually get HIV because a condom broke. Rather, it's usually *I did some risky behavior,* and the thing is, what's behind that risky behavior? Self-hatred? Addiction? See it as an opportunity to change and grow. Your life can just begin."

STIs

SHAINA At some point in their lives, an estimated 80 percent of sexually active people contract HPV.

JULIA I've gone to CityMD so many times to get checked. Any mysterious bump down there—I go!

SHAINA It's good to be cautious.

There's a lot more condomless sex in the gay community because of PrEP [pre-exposure prophylaxis]. At the same time, we have to get tested for everything else every three months. **So everyone is getting tested more frequently than before, and I think they're catching and treating things earlier.**

I'm on PrEP. I don't even ask my partners if they're HIV-positive, because for me it's irrelevant. Guys who are HIV-positive know it and are on a treatment. That means they are undetectable. The levels of HIV in their blood are so low that it's impossible for them to transmit the virus. I have sex with HIV-positive guys, and it's no issue.

I went a little crazy after going on PrEP. There's this one place on Fire Island called Dick Dock. I went there newly on PrEP. I was bent over a railing and had sex with twelve men in the course of two hours. After guy after guy ejaculates into you, there's more lubricant, so it's easier and easier. A cum dump. It was liberating. As a gay man growing up in the AIDS era, I never had that feeling before.

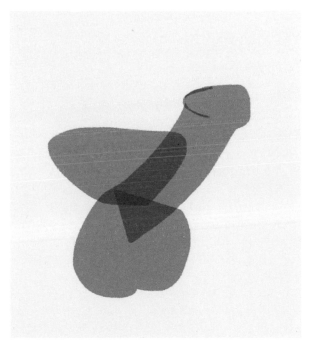

Tio Cuchillos

I've slept with more than seventy-five people. I always use a condom—girlfriend, fiancée, one-night stand, whatever. I'm not gonna play with my health.

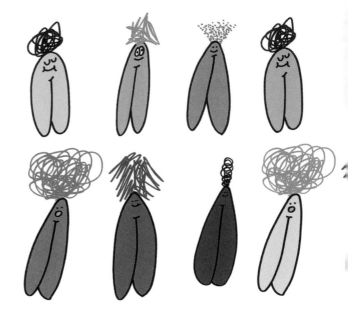

I got infected with herpes when I was twenty-six by my boyfriend. He had herpes on his lip and went down on me. We didn't think about it, and then it was there on my vagina. I went to the ob-gyn and felt gross. And my boyfriend felt bad. **I didn't have an outbreak again until a year later, and then it never came back.**

More than a decade later, I was with a different boyfriend and we were traveling in Costa Rica together. We passed this butterfly museum and it was called the *herbarium* or something like that, so I made a joke about herpes. He quickly mentioned he'd had a big herpes scare when he was eighteen. Somehow later that night it came up again at dinner. He mentioned it was a really big deal for him, where he obsessed over whether he had herpes and looked up all this stuff about it online and felt dirty. (He had tested positive for herpes, but it was a false positive or something.)

In that moment, I stupidly decided to tell him about what happened to me eleven years ago. He got really upset. He said I had made him vulnerable to it and should have told him that happened before we started sleeping together unprotected. It was really awkward and weird, because we were stuck on this vacation together with this tension.

At night, when he tried to have sex with me, I stopped him and said, "Are you sure? Do you feel uncomfortable now because I told you about that herpes thing?"

He said, "Well, actually, I don't know."

That *I don't know* bothered me. But we still had sex, and the rest of the trip was good.

When we got back from the trip, I went to my ob-gyn and asked if herpes was dormant in me. It had been over ten years, but I wanted to be sure I couldn't really give it to him. The doctor said it was still possible, but highly unlikely because I hadn't had a flare-up in so long. But since it never leaves your system, it wasn't *im*possible.

I told my boyfriend that night on the phone. It was the day after we had said *I love you* for the first time. **I thought we had made this new step in our relationship, but he got really upset all over again and told me I had put his health in danger—that I should have told him about it.** Also, I hadn't told him I had HPV [human papillomavirus], because everyone has that and it just didn't cross my mind.

A few days later, he broke up with me. It was terrible. I felt like a bad person because I hadn't told him. Also, I felt dirty. He broke my heart in many ways. What's nice is that two years later, I was dating this new guy, and I mentioned all of it because I didn't want to ever feel that way again. And he said, "Okay, whatever. Everyone has everything—we're humans, we get things. Don't worry. Let's just be safe." He destigmatized all of it for me.

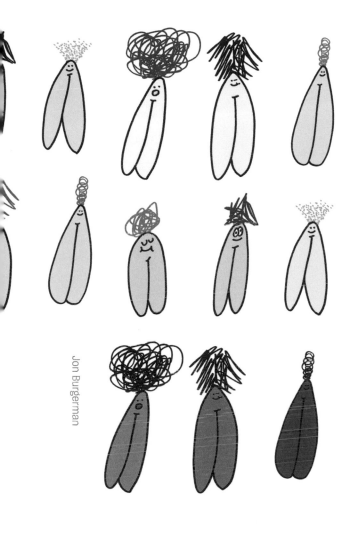

Jon Burgerman

I was a virgin until I was forty-two. I never discussed it with anyone because I was so terribly ashamed. I had never been able to use a tampon, but I couldn't figure out why. I also avoided having my first gynecological exam for a long time. (If I couldn't insert a tampon, how the hell was a metal speculum going to fit?!)

At age twenty-three, after fooling around with a guy and feeling extreme pain, I finally went to a gynecologist and was told I had an imperforate hymen. I had surgery to fix it. The surgery was fairly quick and easy, but it involved stitches and was painful for a few days. In hindsight, I think I avoided sex after that because I was so terrified of feeling more pain. I dated every now and then, but I was so scared of telling a guy about my situation and about my inexperience that I never made it past three dates.

Finally, at forty-one I decided I had to try sex at least once to see what all the fuss was about—and to see if it was even possible for me. After six months on a dating app, I met a wonderful guy who I got along with really well. I felt so at ease with him and decided I would sleep with him. And it was great—it was fabulous!

It was a bit of a shock to me that I was able to have sex finally, never mind enjoy it. We'd been together ten months when he broke up with me. It seemed a little odd, because it came out of nowhere. At a routine doctor's appointment the following month, I was got the shock of my life: I was told I had contracted HPV genital warts. I texted the guy; he didn't respond. I called and emailed him; he didn't answer. When I finally heard from him five months later, he denied it. But I know he was lying, because I had since realized that I saw one singular tiny bump on his penis one time. My gut told me that something was a little bit off, but unfortunately I didn't say anything or ask him about it—I didn't want to embarrass him.

So that's how I got an STI. Life goes on and you can't change the past, but I hope my story helps someone else out there feel less shame.

A lot of lesbians don't talk about protection. When I first came out, I was hyper-paranoid and went to the gyno all the time. I would bring a dental dam on a date and try to eat someone out using it, but it was way too thick. So I understand why people don't use them, but I did.

I was once with a partner for a year. She had HPV [human papillomavirus], so I used the dental dam the whole time. A lot of the women I hook up with now have never even seen a dental dam; I'm introducing them to it. Nowadays I use a dental dam for clit on clit—and I like clit on clit the most—but not for eating out, because it is really thick.

I tested positive for HPV
after a routine Pap smear.
A few years later I developed
genital warts on my external
genitalia. They weren't itchy,
but they were visible to the
eye. I was embarrassed. I went
to the gyno to confirm. I decided
to have a procedure where they
froze them off. It was really
painful. But the pain didn't
last long, and it made them
go away. And that was it. Now
I haven't had an irregular
Pap smear for the past ten years.

I was born in 1971 and came of sexual age when the AIDS crisis was hitting the gay community hard. When I started to act out on my sexual urges, I stayed away from anything I considered dangerous—especially anal sex, even with a condom. For decades I never pursued anal sex; I considered it absolutely forbidden because I associated it with HIV and AIDS.

I started dating my current boyfriend in 2011, and we started to have unprotected sex. I was okay with it, but I could never fully enjoy it and wasn't used to it. One day in 2015 I met a hot man in a porn kino and was so turned on that I fucked him raw (without a condom). This became a regular thing in our weekly meetings, and I started to get concerned about HIV. I contacted a doctor and they informed me about PrEP and gave me a prescription.

Once I started taking PrEP, I went crazy—not only with that guy but with other men as well. I was having all types of unprotected, raw sex with every hot man that wanted it. I was giving and receiving and swallowing and had multiple partners in one day and even had a few men come inside me. It was exhilarating and fun. I finally understood what it felt like to be a gay man pre-AIDS.

I went on like this for a year or so, keeping track of all my tricks—body descriptions, names, cock sizes, what we did, and how good (or not so good) it was. Sex with my boyfriend improved. One evening my boyfriend told me he had started getting discharges from his penis, and he was concerned: did I have something to tell him? My heart sank and I felt horrible. I'd never felt this bad before in my life. I have never (to my knowledge) passed a sexually transmitted disease to a partner, but my boyfriend tested positive for gonorrhea. It was his first STI ever, but it wouldn't be his last: I gave it to him *twice*.

One in four people with a vagina (and one in five people with a penis) have genital herpes. Condoms don't fully protect against it. It can be transmitted even when there are no symptoms, no sores. For most people with genital herpes, there will never be symptoms at all. It's excluded from most STI test panels because doctors know how common it is. And they prioritize blissful ignorance over the "burden of knowing." Because once you know, you must disclose it to every partner.

I've had genital herpes for three years. **I thought I had a patch of razor burn, and the only reason I got tested was because the glands in my neck were tender, like there was a viral cold coming on.** I knew from educating myself about STIs that that was unusual. It turned out to be HSV-1—herpes, type 1, the kind that's usually on the mouth. It was probably transmitted to my vagina via oral sex.

After that little outbreak went away, I never got one again. I completely forget that I even have it for months at a time. And when I remember, it's just a second of, *Oh yeah*. And then the thought drifts away and I forget again.

It isn't a big deal. If you have herpes, don't let anyone tell you it's a big deal. Don't let anyone make you feel like shit about it. There's a one in five chance they have it too, after all. Fuck the stigma. When it comes to navigating sex and love in my twenties, herpes is the least of my worries.

I was with my new boyfriend, painting signs for the Women's March, when I got a text: "This is an anonymous service letting you know that a past sexual partner of yours has tested positive for a sexually transmitted infection. You should go get tested."

My first thought was that it was spam. But then I looked up the service online and it was legit, and I started to panic. **I was always careful and used condoms with people I wasn't in a long-term thing with. But I thought it had to be bad if I was getting this message.** I started shaking and shivering. I was worried about my new boyfriend more than myself—that I had gotten something and given it to him.

My boyfriend was so calm. We talked about the repercussions of each of the STIs. He held me all night. As soon as CityMD opened the next morning, we went together and got rapid HIV tests and full blood testing for everything else. When the HIV test came back negative, I relaxed. A few days later we got our other results: both of us were totally clean.

That experience sucked, but I learned so much about my boyfriend that day. I can't say I would have been as sweet and supportive as he was if the roles had been reversed. We had only been dating a few months, but I think I really fell in love with him that day.

I don't inherently like sex. There's that gross saying, *Sex is like pizza—when it's bad, it's still pizza.*

But sex and pizza both make me feel like shit. I've been trying to figure out why, but I don't have a definitive answer. A lot of it is wrapped up in OCD, specifically surrounding contamination and responsibility. *Contamination* because I was scared into living in a world where STIs were a judgment upon people and a life sentence—that if I were ever to contract an STI, nobody would want to be with me again.

I understand this to be bullshit, but even when I was no longer a middle schooler indoctrinated in that belief system, the fear really persisted—most acutely, the fear of contracting genital herpes. It was based on stories that friends would tell: that you could have sex only with the person you were with when you got it. It's all vestiges of *The Scarlet Letter.* The weird thing about a phobia is it's irrational. To physically be with someone was to expose myself to contracting an STI—HPV, herpes, HIV.

Additionally there's the *responsibility* component. A lot of STIs are asymptomatic. What if I have something and I'm not disclosing it because I don't know I have it? There's the fear that I'm going to get an STI, or give someone an STI I don't know I have. I know those both go beyond the rational.

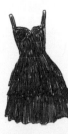

What Does Jessica Rabbit Have That I Don't?

by REBEKAH TAUSSIG

Maybe it would be useful to know that when I was a five-year-old girl, lying alone in the dark, I invented ways to twist my pink Care Bear nightie into a sexy outfit. I knew what *sexy* looked like because I'd seen Jessica Rabbit, and the way her matching sultry eyes and mountain breasts made everyone around her stop, stare, and drool. I'd also spent many secret hours in the basement watching my grandmother's taped "programs" (read: countless episodes of *As the World Turns,* recorded on stacks of VHS tapes), full of muscly men gazing at women in their stilettos and silky blouses. He wanted her, and I wanted that. I wanted to be

sexy—seen as a beautiful object—worth keeping around just to look at. It hadn't occurred to me yet that my paralyzed legs might have an effect on that dream.

It was a Saturday afternoon later that summer (or was it the next summer?) when I decided to wear something dazzling to the library. I put on my blue and white floral dress-up gown—the one overwhelmed by ruffles and lace, of course—and felt regal as my dad pushed me over the bumpy sidewalks. I was a princess riding an elephant, tilting my chin up with a graceful smile. I can still run my fingers over the feeling—I was *beautiful*.

Before we saw the boys, we heard their wild-boy sounds, joking back and forth on their front porch. I prepared myself to be admired. They would certainly catch their breaths at the sight of my splendor. As my dad pushed me past, I couldn't bring myself to look at their smitten expressions; I only heard their chatter disappear. I imagined their eyes transformed into throbbing red hearts as we glided past.

I glowed for the rest of the afternoon, soaring in the revelation that I was one of those girls who made boys stop and stare. As soon as we got home, I flew to my mom, eager to relive the experience with her.

"They couldn't even *speak* as I walked by, Mom. All of them just stared and stared at me." I was bursting. I don't know what she thought in that moment, but I remember her silence. She looked at me, and I saw sadness in her face. In a rush, like a full balloon gushing icy water over my head, I knew. They were not staring at my loveliness. They were staring at my wheelchair.

My sister and I were drinking coffee at the bookstore, feeling bold and independent with her new driver's license. We'd put on fancy black dresses for the occasion. Mine had an extra ruffle around the hem, and I liked the shape of my boobs in it. I could see an older man a few tables over staring in our direction. I pretended not to notice as he stood up and moved closer. "Excuse me," he said, looking at my sister, "I just couldn't help but say, you really should be a model. You're so thin—just stunning." My exquisite sister, already well acquainted with the male gaze at the age of sixteen, tried to deflect. "I think Bekah should be a model!" she said, stroking my hair. "*She's* stunning." I looked away, knowing what was coming next. The guy wasn't deterred. "No, you're thinner," he said to her. "You're just *gorgeous*."

Did I wish the man had aimed his attention at me? Not exactly. Did I cherish my escape from his attention? I did not. I also feel compelled to tell you—and why, I really don't know—I should

keep this to myself—except maybe it's an important piece—that I was wildly jealous of my sister's ability to put on a little dress and make the room stop, stare, and drool, Jessica Rabbit–style.

I am a grown-ass woman in her thirties. I know that reducing someone to an object you ogle in a bookstore is a bad thing. I can also see that desexualization comes with some perks—it can be a bonus, a shield, a superpower of sorts. Like an old lady or a pet, no one worries about their person-of-romantic-interest spending too much time around me. My body is neither threat nor tease nor distraction. No one will punish me for refusing to reciprocate their flirtatious advances. All outcomes that make some parts of life easier. I wonder, though—it's scandalous, I know, but sometimes I *do*—I wonder, for good or bad, what it would have done for my developing understanding of my place in the world—my understanding of myself as a woman among women—my connection to my own self, sensuality, sexuality, sex—had my body been reduced to a sexual object, too.

Once, when moving down the main drag of my small college town with a group of friends, a man shouted at me on the street, "You're the hottest girl in a wheelchair I've ever seen!"

I rolled my eyes, kept moving, and smiled to myself. The man hollering at me on the street was loud, drunk, and thoughtless, but he did not make me feel small or powerless like the man who, unprovoked, approached me from behind, grabbed the handlebars on my chair, and pushed me up a long ramp in front of the library. "There you go!" he said cheerily when we reached the top—convinced, I'm sure, he'd met his good-deed quota for the month. I'm not routinely objectified as a sex object, but I do know the weight of objectification. It's just that I'm categorized as a different sort of object—a signifier of brokenness, helplessness, always in need of some friendly assistance. The moment on the street with the drunk man was fleeting, and I grabbed hold of it like a late-summer firefly.

When I eventually did find a man who stared at my body like an ice cream cone, I leaped at the chance to be lustily devoured. *Finally*—verification that I am valuable, wanted. This must be what it feels like to belong. I hovered somewhere above, watching him watch me. I studied the desire/pleasure on his face while he consumed me, as I tried to quiet the spasms in my legs, striving for a scene worthy of *As the World Turns*.

It didn't make me feel like I'd always imagined Jessica Rabbit felt when she sauntered in her red dress with the slit up the side. His gaze didn't taste sweet and bright; it was sour and stale. I didn't feel floaty and light; I felt heavy and nauseous. Even so, it took me a very long time to let go of being wanted by him. This had to be better than nothing at all, right? I started wearing big baggy shirts to bed and pretending to be asleep when he got off work.

I knew it as a continuum—a spectrum—everything operating in the space between desexualization and sexual objectification, between infantilization and ogling. I'd already memorized the equation: sexy → sex = value. The rules and patterns, expectations and goals were pre-programmed and unending. I saw them play out in the soaps and cartoons, on the streets and the covers of magazines lining the checkout counter, on the faces of men watching my sister. I wished to be off the scale that found me wanting—left me wanting—like I wished for world peace. Wouldn't that be nice.

When we first meet, you throw me off course. I can't find you in my numbers or charts. You're humming somewhere in the ether, existing outside the parameters I've always known. When we move through a crowd, sit face-to-face over doughnuts, snuggle side by side in bed, I can't catch your gaze in my hands—you're doing something else with your eyes. *What is it?* With you I am perplexed, amazed, disoriented, wide-eyed, peaceful.

The air exhaled from your nose tickles the top of my lip. Your beard is rough against my forehead and the backs of my shoulders. "Can you help me move my legs this way?" I ask. "Let's try this instead," you say. Somehow I'm not thinking about this as a "sex scene" or the ways it might get "messed up," but I still wait for that moment when you see me as an object—*Why won't you just consume me?* I don't think you can help it—you see me as an object *and*. Desire. Pleasure. Heartbeat. Closeness. Preference. Giggles. Voice. If I try to leave my body, you'll notice. The corners of your eyes crinkle as you look into mine. "Why are you smiling?" I ask, looking back.

I am turning forty-two years old this year, and through a mixture of choice and circumstance I have never had a sustained intimate sexual relationship with another person. And yet with genuine honesty, I feel pretty great about my life. I have dozens of beautifully fulfilling relationships, a loving and supportive family, and lots of time to pursue multiple passion projects and create positive contributions to the world. Plus I can give myself a sparkling orgasm in the time it takes to hit the snooze button in the morning and wait for the next alarm to ring.

OVERCOMING THE UNEXPECTED

JULIA We got a shocking number of stories about vaginismus—which is a condition that no one is really talking about.

SHAINA We included only a few of them here, but believe us, we could have made an entire book about vaginismus.

JULIA If you're dealing with this condition, know that there are treatments that can help.

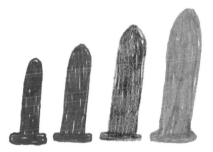

When my mom was in her fifties, I had to show her where her vagina was. She had a hysterectomy, and the doctor gave her antibiotic ointment that had to go up her vagina in order to help it heal inside. She was at home recovering and I was the only one taking care of her. I administered her oral medications and emptied out her catheter when it was full. However, when I saw on her discharge paperwork that she had vaginal medication, I just reminded her she needed to put it up her vagina, then shut her door.

I heard her crying. She called me in and was like, *I...don't know where my vagina is.* I could not believe what I was hearing, but I knew the medication was crucial for her aftercare. So I put all my feelings aside, got a hand mirror, and showed where everything was. But she still couldn't do it. After much deliberation and freaking out from both of us, I had to put the medicine up her vagina.

I had top surgery and a hysterectomy. **I rushed to get my hysterectomy when Trump was elected because he said he was going to cut off transgender rights: I got it in November 2016.** Around the three-month mark, I started having complications. The hysterectomy led to an intestinal prolapse, and I almost died at that point. But they said I was okay to fly, so I flew from San Francisco to JFK—and when I landed I was puking up green stuff. I had to get rushed to the hospital. I spent two weeks in the hospital and lost thirty pounds. I had to figure out how to walk again. It's been two years, and I'm still affected by this.

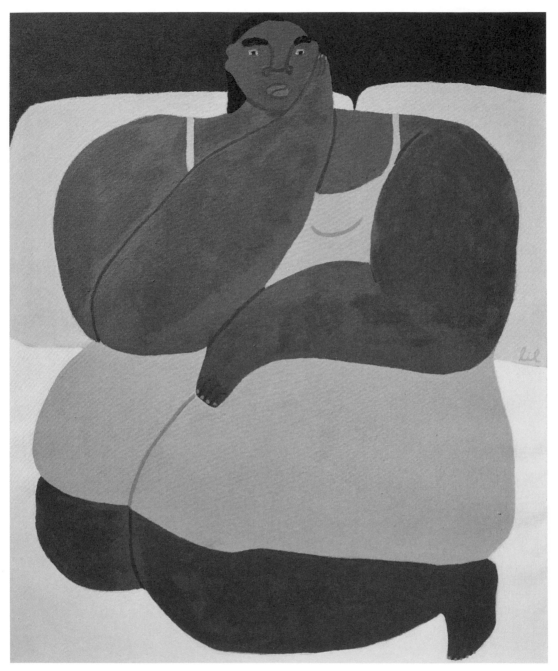

Lilian Martinez

I didn't have sex until I was thirty-four years old. I'm not entirely sure how this happened. I'm a straight cis woman. Sex was *super* not discussed in my [liberal, nonreligious] family. I got my sex ed at my [progressive] Unitarian Universalist Church. I was in high school in the nineties, when all of the messaging was about AIDS and the various other things that could kill you if you had sex. I had crushes on various boys in high school, but none of them wanted to have sex with me, as far as I could tell. There was no dating culture at my college, so I continued not having sex with people.

By the time I was twenty-five or so, not having had sex started seeming so weird that I felt embarrassed about it, and ashamed, and then like some kind of a freak. I dated various great men in my twenties and even slept with them, in the literal sense, but they were too gentlemanly to pressure me and I was too embarrassed to bring up the topic—that I was a virgin, and I was nervous, and I didn't know what to do.

Then suddenly I was in my thirties and still hadn't had sex, and it was something I didn't discuss even with my closest friends. Finally, I met a great guy at thirty-four. He barely blinked when I told him it would be my first time...and then we discovered I had vaginismus, so if he got remotely near my vulva with any part of himself, everything would clench up tighter than, I don't know—what's the analogy?—Thor's fist. Does Thor punch people? Early attempts at penetration were extremely painful. It took months until we were able to have sex

successfully. That lasted a year and a half or so. It was great!

But then my body decided we were done. Honestly, I think my heart had decided we were done. My brain refused to listen, but my vagina was like, *Yep, got the message,* and shut down. We stayed together for a couple more years without sex, and now he is marrying a lovely woman and I am very happy for him. But here I am at forty-three and I've had sex with one guy, and I know my genitals aren't really on board with the sex thing. I get extremely anxious about dating, and I'm intimidated by the idea of bringing up the whole "vagina situation" with a new man, and—ugh, the whole thing just feels fraught and embarrassing and awful.

Weird thing, I still don't discuss this topic with anyone but my BFF (who lost her virginity at like twelve and had a lot of sex before marrying in her early twenties). But I suspect some of my close friends are in similar situations. I had one brief conversation with a very old friend lately where we worked out that, yeah, our pelvic regions have similar situations, except *she's* still a virgin at forty-four.

It makes me wonder how common this is. In a culture that goes on about sex so dang much, it feels countercultural and, yes, shameful to be having no sex. We certainly don't go around telling anyone we aren't getting any. (Or blaming men for not sleeping with us—I'm looking at you, incels.) It's a weird secret and I don't like it, and by the way I'm a writer—but I've never written about it.

Until now.

I decided to stay a virgin until my marriage. Then when I had my first experience, he couldn't enter my vagina. We tried again a couple of times and we couldn't. I started to think there's something wrong with me. I told my friends about it, and they said they had a friend with the same problem—it's called *vaginismus.*

When you grow up in a culture where sex is taboo and you can't talk about it, when you want to have a sexual experience, your muscles contract and don't allow you to do it. It's an unconscious problem. You can't control your body. So now I have started to see a hypnotist; I've had three sessions.

When I went to a doctor before all this, she tried to insert her dilator but couldn't. That's when she screamed at me, "What's wrong with you?" But I didn't know what it was called then, and I was too ashamed to tell her that I couldn't have sex with my husband, so I just started to cry and left her office. Now I am doing exercises to control my breath and my body. I also look at pictures of vaginas—I'm supposed to look at them and say, *I have a vagina, and it's okay for my husband to enter it.*

I am Moroccan, and sex is taboo. I am thankful that my husband understands. And my friends' friend who had this same problem? She is cured—and is pregnant now! It's a long road to a cure, but it happens.

I don't know if I'm the only person in the same dilemma I'm in. I've only recently started having what I consider to be good sex. I'm bisexual. I've never had an orgasm before—never. I've been with many different kinds of partners: men, women, trans folk. **I don't know if it's something with my biology, or it's mental.** I can get into it, but it just never gets there.

I thought by this time it would have happened. Maybe the fact that I keep wanting it to happen psychs me out? I'm just not that sensitive down there—that's the thing (even if it's me to me, or my partner to me). When I try by myself, I guess I'm not in the right mindset. The closest I ever got was with my current partner.

It's not like I've ever had horrible sex; I've always had decent sex. I used to sleep with men a lot. It was always about just getting to the bedroom and having fun, and enjoying the person on an intimate level, but now I have the emotional aspect, too. But it sits in the back of my mind, despite how much I enjoy being in the bedroom with her. I always prefer to make it more about her—I want her to have fun. So for all the people out there who've never had an orgasm, know that you are not alone.

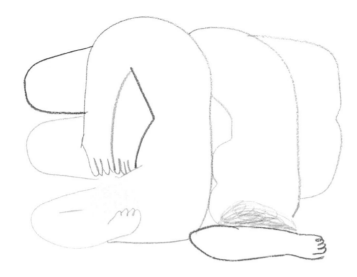

Ohni Lisle

I've got a bag of shit stuck to my stomach, over a few inches of small intestine that pokes out of my belly like a penis. It's called an ileostomy, and it's how I go to the toilet. It can be hard to feel sexy knowing your shit bag is there—most people aren't confronted with their intestines on a daily basis! So when it comes to having sex, I also have to share this new body of mine with my partner.

Before I had my ileostomy surgery, I asked him if he would freak out and feel disgusted when it came to having sex once I got my stoma. He said he hoped not, but he wouldn't know until I had it done. I did worry about this a lot, hoping it wouldn't kill our sex life, hoping it would be something we could work on together. Thankfully, he wasn't bothered by it.

You can only see the bag stuck to my stomach; my stoma is not visible unless I remove the bag. My partner is not interested in seeing my stoma itself. Initially I was hurt by this—until he said, "I don't want to see it not because I don't care, but because I don't show you my arsehole! It's the same thing."

So, back to sex. I've found that it helps me mentally get in the mood if I empty my stoma bag beforehand; that way I don't feel the weight of shit hanging on my stomach while I'm having sex. I also have special intimacy knickers designed specifically for ostomates. They are high-waisted, with an internal pocket that my stoma bag sits in to keep it secure, and there is a slit in the crotch so you can have penetrative sex without taking them off. I wore these like protective armor every time we had sex for the first few months, worrying that without them I wouldn't feel sexy or look attractive to my partner. Then I decided to take the plunge and not put them on. I wanted to have sex with my bag on show, not held down and covered by material.

I held my breath, waiting for the sound of disgust from my partner. I'd grossly misjudged him—of course he didn't react like that! He was not interested in the slightest that I had my shit bag; he still found me attractive, and most of all he still wanted to have sex.

Since then, I've stopped worrying about my stoma bag when we have sex. I do sometimes still wear my intimacy knickers because I feel sexy in them, but I don't hide behind them anymore. Everyone shits—we all have intestines inside us. I'm just a bit different in how mine work, but it isn't anything to be ashamed of. I can still feel sexy, attractive, and confident with an ileostomy. Sex can still be fun, loving, adventurous, fast, slow—whatever you want it to be.

Because of our faith, my now-husband, then–college boyfriend and I were convinced that sex before marriage was wrong. **In the three and a half years we dated before getting married, we would passionately kiss and leave each other's dorm rooms in a hot and horny daze, but with our "purity" safely in check.** We were footloose and intercourse-free, with heart eyes and curiosity about what sex would be like. I couldn't wait.

I remember this time period as both torturous and thrilling. The day we got engaged was our first time totally undressing and lying in bed together. No penis-in-vagina, but we would masturbate with each other. It started to feel like we were drifting into the realm of wrong. I remember feeling so much shame during that time, which makes me sad for my young self. We were freaking engaged and twenty-one and loved each other—*and* our hormones were out of control.

A few months before our wedding, I went to the gynecologist for the first time to get birth control and be examined before the big *I Do* and *Doing It*. As she inserted the metal dilator inside me and began to open it, I almost passed out from the pain; she had to switch to the pediatric size, which opened but was still tight. She told me gently that it could help to use my fingers to try stretching my vagina before my wedding night. I did that, but it was so painful. I began to feel nervous about sex—maybe it wasn't what it was cracked up to be. Couldn't we just keep foreplaying forever?

The wedding night came after a beautiful and fun day. We drove, exhausted, to our bed-and-breakfast, and I slipped into my special white lingerie. Sexy clothing lasted for the requisite five seconds before my husband stripped it off. It wasn't long before it was time to seal the deal, and I thought I was ready. He put it in, or so I thought, and the pain was excruciating. I began to weep. I learned he had only put the tip in. This was devastating. I couldn't take it. We proceeded for the next fifteen or so minutes to get it in. I cried, and he reassured me, "Babe, it's okay. This is just how it goes." I cried harder

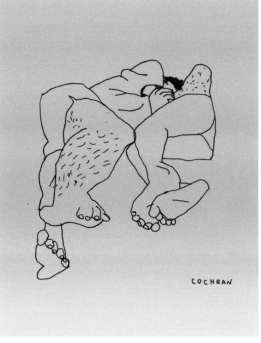

Josh Cochran

because I thought he meant, "Sorry, this is just how sex is." When I told him that's what I thought, he exclaimed, "No, no! I meant that it's okay, you're totally normal. This is normal first-time sex. I'm not expecting anything different."

He finally got his penis all the way in (though it was by no means a boner anymore), and I asked him if we could lie just like that for a while. It was too painful when he moved, but I thought maybe that would help me stretch out some. We lay in each other's arms, him inside me, me silently crying while he soothed me. After a bit, he came out, I bled, and he held me. I'm still not sure if it was technically sex—he never came—but it was a special night.

Eight years later, we've got it figured out. He's still my only sexual partner, and though I no longer subscribe to the idea that everyone should save themselves for marriage (unless they just want to), I'm glad we've gotten to learn together how to have sex. We're pretty damn good at it, in my opinion. Then again, who really knows?

I've had sexsomnia throughout my entire sexual adulthood for twenty-plus years. While asleep, not consciously, I will initiate sex with the person I'm in bed with. It's like another form of sleepwalking. Different things have happened as a result.

Usually my partner has been totally fine with it, and we have sex. Other times I've woken up during sex and been like, *Ugh, this is weird. I'm tired, I'm not going to finish doing this.* And then we go back to sleep. Women have been jealous because I talk dirty, which I don't usually do when I'm awake. They think I'm thinking of somebody else. They will try to catch me and say, "I know you were sleeping, so who were you thinking about?" Other women were offended because it felt super-rapey. I can be very aggressive, apparently. In the morning they call me a "fucking asshole," and I don't even know what I did! I can only apologize, because I remember just bits and pieces of it.

Even when I knew my partner well, I think the forcefulness scared them. It's a terrible feeling to know you're doing that. It hasn't happened in many years, but it happened recently with my new girlfriend for the first time. I grabbed her in the middle of the night. She hit me to stop me, and she said I stood up and just looked at her—or "through her," in that creepy sleepwalking way—and then went back to bed. The next day, she was laughing hysterically about it. She said it was so weird and she can't believe it happened. But I had told her ahead of time that I do this. **I definitely prepare women for it if I'm sleeping in a bed with them.** Actually, another woman I was dating last year was looking forward to it, but it never happened.

It wasn't like I was ever sexually repressed. I always had a healthy sex life, and sex-positive partners. I could never figure out why it happened. I think maybe it has something to do with eating sugar before bed, because I used to do that a lot, and when I did it the other night, it happened again.

I'm twenty-eight, dating guys I meet online, and every time a guy tries to kiss me and I decline, I say, "It's been a long time."

Actually, it's been *no* time; I'm a kissing virgin and a virgin-virgin.

I'm just now getting all my seventeen-year-old firsts in: hand-holding, cuddling, masturbation. I grew up Catholic, and I always blamed it on that. But that's not quite it. **Something in my body feels excruciatingly vulnerable when it comes to being physical with another person, and I'm still not sure what that's about.**

The guy I'm seeing right now is the first ever to ask me if it was okay to hold my hand, touch me, kiss me. When he does that, at least one part of the mystery is solved for me: I need to consent—*enthusiastically,* as they say—to everything. Because physical touch is not easy for me at all, but I'm still human and I still need it. I just need to be asked. Some people think that's lame and unromantic. The movies portray straightforward communication as something two conspiratorial virgins might do before their first time. But ambiguity is not sexy. Not for me; I think it's dangerous.

So I'm trying to remain celibate for many reasons beyond those of religion. But my therapist had a frank conversation with me about what I am willing to do. "Lack of communication and consent," she said, "can often lead to date rape." But consent and communication aren't just *necessary* for me, I've discovered; communication turns me on.

When one of my dates grabbed me in a dark alley wordlessly and pulled me close, I felt like a helpless little thing. I had no control and no power. "Not here," was all I said, and I felt so much shame. But my body had overridden any work that my brain could have done in that moment to decide if I wanted to kiss this person or not. The absence of honest communication, of any words at all, shut me down and turned me right off.

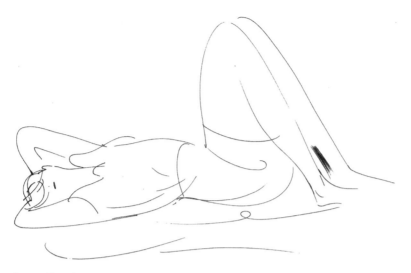

Roman Muradov

A few years ago, after a very long dry spell, I started dating a new guy. And to get to the point—sex was painful. Not extremely painful, but always uncomfortable. Not good. This was really problematic. I kept hoping it would get better—that maybe I just had to get more comfortable with him, or that it was all in my head. But it didn't. After we broke up, I went to the gynecologist hoping she would be able to figure out what was wrong, but she said everything looked normal. I thought I would just be doomed forever, that I would never be able to make a relationship work.

A while later, listening to a random podcast, the narrator started talking about pelvic-floor-muscle problems and how she went to a physical therapist who was able to help. After doing some research, I made an appointment with a physical therapist who specialized in that sort of thing. It was a strange experience, but the therapist was really nice and made me feel as comfortable as possible. Basically, my pelvic-floor muscles were tensed up, and at the appointments she put her fingers inside me and pressed on the different muscles to stretch them out

and help them relax. This was not pleasurable, but it felt the same as when any other muscle is tight and you press on it to try to relieve the pain. There were exercises to help strengthen other abdominal muscles that were supposed to be working better so the pelvic-floor muscles wouldn't be engaged improperly to compensate. I ended up going once a week for three or four months.

My homework was to get a set of vaginal dilators of increasing sizes. A few times a week, I had to insert one and leave it in for ten minutes while doing deep-breathing exercises. As the therapy progressed, I moved up one size every few weeks. And when I finally started dating someone new, it had worked: sex was no longer uncomfortable.

That relationship didn't work out either, but it was such a relief not to feel like a freak. It's upsetting that a highly recommended gynecologist didn't know about this, or think to suggest such an obvious possibility. That if I hadn't randomly heard about it, I might have gone my whole life with a problem that was not just about physical pain but a barrier to being able to make a normal human connection.

SEX LITERACY

ERICA CHIDI COHEN

My name is Erica Chidi Cohen. I am a doula, health educator, and author. I am also the cofounder and CEO of LOOM, which exists to empower people as they navigate their sexual, reproductive, and parenting experience. Basically, it is helping people advocate for their own well-being.

My parents are both from the clinical field—my dad was a doctor and my mom was a nurse—and I was always really fascinated by their work. There was always a lot of room for inquiry in my house, and because my parents had clinical backgrounds, they would infuse the subject of sex, say, with medical context.

Since I was young—and because my parents had the background they had—people would always ask me about things that had to do with their bodies. I was the go-to person for on-the-fly sex-ed and body questions. Eventually I found my way to reproductive health as a career, and that definitely stems from my parents.

I started off my career in the Bay Area as a founding member of a non-profit organization called The Birth Justice Project. Our focus was helping pregnant people incarcerated in the San Francisco jail to get childbirth education during their pregnancy, doula support during their labor, and postpartum help after they gave birth. The big takeaway for me was that no matter what you're going through—whether you're in jail or the CEO of a tech startup—your need for information is very much the same. So beyond the economic component, everybody needs support. And everybody had the same questions: people wanted to know how to keep their baby safe. And people who were having their first baby were scared. That's what I discovered during my time with that organization—that everyone just wanted information.

Out of that, I realized that pregnancy, periods, sex, and menopause are universal experiences for people across the board. These experiences are great equalizers. Everyone has the same basic needs; we forget that a lot. That is the standpoint I work from.

I've been teaching a sex class at LOOM for a year. The first time I shared the curriculum, I saw how much it resonated with people. We are taught to evaluate our sexual proficiency through the partners we're with, as opposed to having a deeper understanding of what we actually like ourselves. And seeing that in action was an aha moment for me. Every time I shared that statement in the class—that we can shift how we come at our own sexual experiences—I could feel a deep breath in the room, and I realized how much more we need to be validating women in their own personal sexual experiences. We need to be empowering them to decipher their own likes and needs separate from the likes and needs of others.

In my field, I deal a lot with abortion and miscarriage. And it's really important that we see both abortion and miscarriage as pregnancy-related experiences. I think when we divorce them from that original departure point, it creates an uncomfortable hierarchy. Of course, a person moving through an abortion and someone moving through a miscarriage are coming at it from two very different emotional places: in the first case someone has to make a decision, whereas in the second it's a natural physiological event that the body will start if a pregnancy is not viable. But the compassion has to be anchored in the fact that both of these outcomes started in the same place, and that either person is going through some kind of physical loss—the body is losing contents. So if we can look at it like that, rather than from a dogmatic or religious perspective, it allows people to have compassion for someone. This person was pregnant and now they are not. It's a physical loss, and it's not comfortable. If we look at it this way, it can help us to show up for people and be compassionate for them.

There is a lot of ignorance around menopause—to be menopausal, you have to not have your period for an entire calendar year. And when it comes to menopause, it should be dealt with prophylactically; you can't be learning about it while you go through it. Especially because perimenopause—the period of time leading up to menopause—can last ten years. So we really need to be getting ahead of that and learning about it in advance. Unfortunately, the patriarchy makes it hard for us to have more clarity around that experience.

This entire area—sex education, menstruation, menopause—feels very neglected in our culture. One of the most common questions I get is: *Is my period normal?* There are a lot of questions about normalcy. *Is it normal to be this color? Are "period poops" normal? Should I be feeling this way?* There's a major knowledge deficit for women around their reproductive health and their sexual literacy. I'm amazed at how much people have to ask

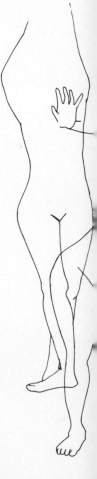

because there is such a fundamental lack of information available. And I think it's due to how much the patriarchy dictates our existence. In most countries, obviously, but definitely in the United States.

It would be great if people could get really good sex education while they're in school, but the possibility of that is currently pretty low. So as people get older and they still lack the information they need, they get curious and reach out for information. And that's where places like LOOM come in. And now there are a lot of great books people can reach for: *Taking Charge of Your Fertility, Heavy Flow, Come as You Are,* and many others.

There's a lot of newer material out there to help with building this knowledge, but first people need to be curious. You know, you're born with the hardware in your body, but you have to keep fine-tuning that hardware. People think they know all about sex, but there is so much to learn. It's about not being afraid to get on that journey—and to continue that journey toward body literacy.

This notion of *body literacy* was developed by two midwives in Canada, Geraldine Matus and Laura Wershler. They started the Justisse Method in 1987, which focuses on helping people develop the skills to practice fertility awareness—a form of contraception that can also help a person conceive. Body literacy, at its core, is being able to observe the reproductive functions in your body—when you're bleeding vaginal secretions, for example, or what your body temperature is. It's about recording this information and making some kind of narrative based on that information so you have a cognitive awareness of the physiological events going on in your body. For so many people, that awareness doesn't exist. Either they aren't really engaging with their body or perhaps they've been on a hormonal birth control that stops that kind of physiological communication between the ovaries and the pituitary gland, so they lack a true understanding of how their body works. And it's important for people to gain this understanding—it's really about learning how your body functions and taking a more active role in how your body works.

Another important term is *sex positivity,* which means feeling good about wherever you are on the sexual experience spectrum—whether you're having lots of sex with multiple partners, or having sex only with yourself, or not having sex at all. It's really about celebrating and reinforcing wherever you're at, so long as you feel safe and comfortable. And it's about having empathy for yourself and curiosity around those sexual experiences. It's not about having a hierarchy around what is considered sexual or what is considered "positive sexual behavior." The idea is that you've already started and it's just about developing compassion for yourself as your journey continues. The hardest part for so many people is developing more compassion for themselves and anchoring themselves in their own sexual experiences, not in those of others.

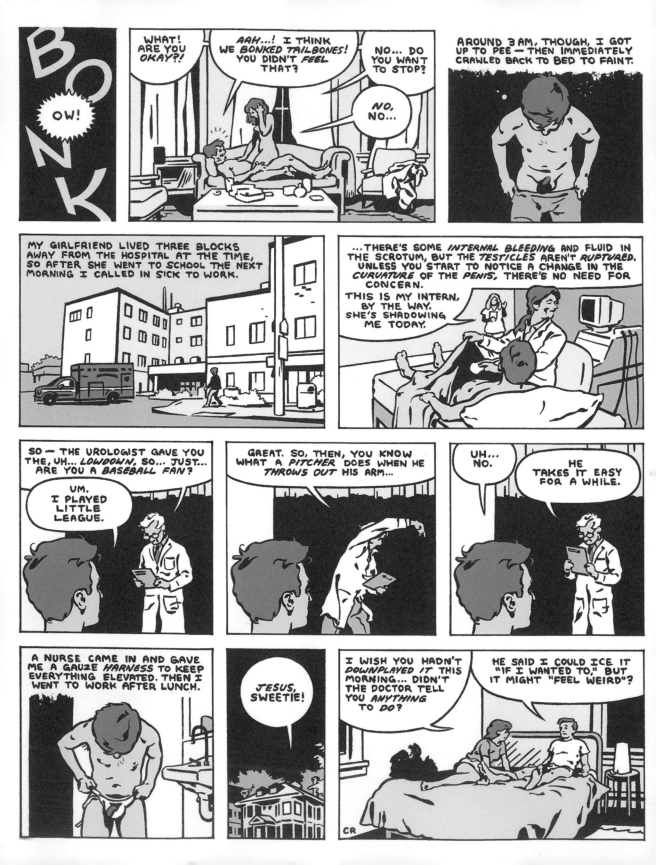

WHOOPS! WHAT???

Casey Roonan

SHAINA We've heard lots of stories of queefs during sex.

JULIA Who hasn't queefed during sex?

SHAINA True. At least queefs don't smell bad.

Farting during sex is funny. I've definitely been going down on a girl and she completely farted in my face. She was embarrassed and I just kept going. What's the point in pointing it out if it's already done?

The first condom I bought was an "extended pleasure" condom, because I was like *I don't want to come too early.* And they have this numbing agent in them. So I was gonna have sex with my girlfriend for the first time, and I opened the condom with my mouth. And a few seconds later I was like, *Why are my lips numb?* **Then I put it on, and I couldn't feel anything down there.** I was like, *What a calamity this is!*

My partner was masturbating, but called me over because he wanted to finish in my mouth. He ended up coming just as I was leaning over, and the cum shot up into my nose. **I had to blow my nose so much to get it all out!**

I met this guy once who had beads under the skin of his penis. It's almost like a dermal piercing, but it's in the penis. **At first I thought there was something crazy wrong with his penis, but it felt amazing.**

I was dating this awesome girl, and we were waiting for the Long Island Rail Road. Her family had had a barbecue, but the food turned up my stomach; I had the bubble guts. When she dropped me at the train, we started to make out. **Then I started to eat her out, but the train came so I rushed for it.** I went to the bathroom because I precame. I had shit stains in my drawers!

I've had anal-sex moments that were gross. Like one time, she said she was ready for it. We talked about it, and then I went for it, and there was no way I could get in—the head of my dick instantly hit fecal matter. Maybe she wasn't that experienced. **But if you're backed up, it's gonna make a mess.**

The first girl I dated in high school, we didn't do much at all. We would just make out for a really long time. I would finger her, and that was the most that ever happened. There was never any interest shown in my penis. It was frustrating. Then I started dating another girl right before my senior year. The second or third time we hung out, she started giving me a hand job. I couldn't believe that someone was touching my penis, so I didn't say anything when it started to hurt. She was grabbing it lightly, so her hand was moving up and down over it, but it wasn't stimulating anything. She was jerking me off the way you jerk someone off when you have lube, but there was no lube. So she was going really fast and rough.

I was immediately turned off, but not enough to lose my erection, because nobody had ever touched my penis before. She asked, "Is this good?" and I didn't know how to explain to her how to do it better. It was becoming so uncomfortable and there was no way I would come from it. So I said, "Oh yeah—I'm going to come!" I got up and put my dick in a sock and pretended to come.

The next day, I had plans to go with a friend to the zoo. We took the train in, but it was impossible for me to walk around because my dick was so chafed. It would rub against my leg and irritate it. So I was limping across the zoo. My friend, who didn't have much experience with women, was furious with me.

He said, "You don't know what you have!" And I said, "I do. And it hurts."

This story starts with a very attractive black guy—huge dick—and ends with $110,000 in insurance billing.

I had never seen anything this monstrous—which had never been a problem. It was New Year's Eve and I had popped by a sex party before going to the Eagle, and I ended up having sex with him there. I remember I was on the ground. There was a TV and a sofa, and gay porn was playing. It was a doggy-style situation. Suddenly something felt unusual. And then very painful. I backed off a bit. I didn't think too much about it.

A week or two later I was lying in bed, trying to fall asleep, when I felt this incredibly sharp pain that went from my rectum and shot up my back. My whole being. It concerned me, but I also thought, *This will go away.* When several weeks had passed and I didn't get better, I went to my high-end anal doctor. He looked at my ass and said I had an anal fissure—a tear. I remember it was a Tuesday. He said, "You have two options for this: you can wait this out and let your body heal, or I'm doing surgery on Friday and I can fit you in to seal it up. That's the quickest recovery."

So I said, "Sure—let's do it." I'd been to him before for a minor back surgery, so I wasn't bothered by the idea. I was in the recovery room afterward, and the doctor comes over and says, "Oh my god, we were all in there—all the nurses and I—and we just felt so bad for you."

Apparently the tear was so big in my rectal wall that they all gasped. He got authorization to put botox in my sphincter because he felt that my rectum was too tight. It was instant relief—no spasms—but the cost was so much. Fortunately my insurance covered most of it. I keep seeing this guy, and I have been tempted again, but then I remember how long it took to heal—six months!

The doctor had me get a training kit of butt plugs—three sizes—so I could stretch it out. He asked if I had a friend who could help me. Ha ha! I said, "No, I don't have a friend who will put butt plugs up me while hanging out drinking wine and watching *Schitt's Creek.*"

I bought the butt plugs, but I never used them.

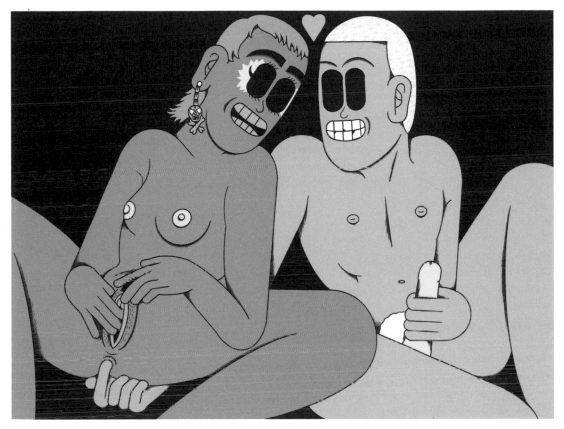

John F. Malta

**I'll never forget the first time I experienced
female ejaculation.**

I was twenty years old, and spending a semester
abroad. I had met a guy at a bar, and we'd been texting and had one date where we engaged in a whole
lot of PDA. Then one weekend my roommate was
away, and I invited him over. We smoked a spliff
and were making out, which led quickly to sex. I
was on top. We both came almost immediately, and
it was the most intense orgasm I'd ever had.

Afterward he said, "I guess you liked that." That's
when I realized the bed was soaking wet. I was kind
of embarrassed, but mostly I felt awesome.

We fucked a bunch more times that night, but
mostly on my roommate's bed—it was drier. I never
told her that, though. Kind of messed up.

I had a girl once call me the wrong name. She was
so drunk. Met her at a bar, walked home stumbling,
and she started calling me Bob or something. I kept
saying, "That's not me. I'm not Bob."

She came to my place and we started making out.
**Then I realized it wasn't fair if we had sex since
she was so drunk.** So we went to sleep. Then in
the morning I said, "Hi, I'm Ethan—do you want an
aspirin?" And I told her she'd been calling me Bob.
And she said, "Oh, shit; that's my ex."

She took the aspirin, and we had a fine morning.
Now she's the drummer in my band.

I was with a coworker and her friend. We were all in our mid-twenties, and I was working behind the counter. We had been drinking steadily and engaging in cheery conversation until the moment my shift was up. I joined the two of them at a table and we continued. **To save money, the friend recommended we go to her apartment for drinks.** Her place was very tasteful and mature—showing all the signs of a serious graduate student—and covered in cat hair. The friend sympathetically offered an allergy medication, which made me drowsy. After a few more rounds of drinks, we decided it was late and time to crash.

After about twenty minutes, I was beckoned over from the living-room couch I'd been assigned for the night. The coworker and her friend had started doing foreplay and wanted me to join in. We made out, licked, fingered, and sucked. But the medication was making it increasingly difficult to perform—I was erect, that was no problem—but I felt desperately sleepy. By the time I was pumping away at the coworker, it was all I could do to stay awake. I just wanted it to be over. Willing myself to finish, I emptied into the condom and rolled over, grateful.

While I caught my breath, the friend asked the coworker, "Did you come?" She said, "Eh—you win some, you lose some." I felt terrible.

It was a Friday night at the Eagle. I was wearing light-gray Lululemon shorts, which are quick drying. I went to the bathroom. I was hooking up with this guy. I turned away to pee and he was behind me. Suddenly I felt this warmth—he was peeing on me!

This was at three in the morning, and all I could think was *I have a flight to San Francisco at seven in the morning, and now my favorite shorts are soaked.* I left the bar quickly. I put the shorts in my bathroom sink and was washing them. An hour or two later—despite the Lululemon claim—they still weren't dry. I still brought them on the plane. **And fortunately I had a window seat, so I line-dried the shorts on the armrest of my seat.** By the time I landed, they were dry; I put them on and went to Dolores Park.

We drove out three hours to go to Sawnee Mountain in Georgia. We were planning to do this really romantic thing. We were talking and it was really nice. **He was very sweet, but he was supernervous.** And the first thing that happened is he just missed my mouth. And then he bit my ear. It started to bleed. It was terrifying. But that was the start of my first time.

In my freshman year at college, I started to go out with a guy. Soon after we started dating, we went back to my dorm room and proceeded to make out. **He pulled down his pants and motioned for me to give him a blow job.** Considering that I had never done that before, I started to blow on his penis! He immediately got up, and that was the end of that!

I was so embarrassed when I learned what I did wrong. Looking back, it would have been much better if he had instructed me.

Roman Muradov

—PARDON MY HARDON.

I am painfully shy and afraid of ever seeming like I don't know what I'm doing. These traits combined on the night I first had sex—with a guy I hardly knew and did not wish to date. I did not want him to know I hadn't had sex before. I was ready to be A Person Who Has Sex. I was on my period and had not removed my tampon, but by the time we were half-naked on his bed it seemed too late, so I just let events play out. Neither of us mentioned it at any point. I forgot to notice how I felt about the sex— I was too busy thinking about digging through my vagina for a tampon string later on.

I dug over the toilet. I dug squatting in the shower. I cried and emailed a professor that I would miss that day's test. I went to the campus nurse and told her I'd been drunk and forgotten if I removed my tampon. She dug—and dug—until she found and retrieved the tampon.

I told my professor about it over wine that night. She said if he was a good guy, he'd send flowers. I did not want flowers. He did not send flowers.

When I was twenty-one, I finally had a boyfriend, Tim, and I felt comfortable enough to have sex for the first time. I left New York for a long weekend to visit him in Colorado, where he was going to school. I think we were both feeling a lot of anticipation around having sex for the first time together (he had had sex before). I got waxed, bought a new bra, and couldn't stop thinking about it—I was finally going to have sex!

In his bedroom, we made out and things started to get steamy. We got undressed. I was so excited! Tim had warned me that he sometimes had issues with getting hard, but I didn't really know how that would impact us. I just saw it as information that made him feel vulnerable, and thus more approachable—and likely more understanding of any issues I had. But he couldn't get hard enough to penetrate me—and when he tried, I queefed! **It was the most embarrassing moment of my life.**

He said, "Whoa!" when it happened, and I just froze. We never tried to have sex again that weekend. I was so sad and disappointed. When I got back to New York, I used a vibrator and broke my hymen. When Tim visited me in New York six weeks later, we had sex. He couldn't believe I was a virgin because I didn't bleed or seem to be in pain. I was so relieved to say I wasn't a virgin anymore.

I must have been about twenty-four—New York, summer of 1999. It was the birthday of my ex-girlfriend, and we had all gone out with friends. Gotten drunk. And despite not wanting to, Maggie somehow talked me into spending the night with her. Or maybe I just needed a place to crash that night, and she offered—I'm not sure.

We were in the back of a taxi on our way back to her place. I didn't really want to sleep with her that night, which she sensed, but she was determined. Her strategy was simple and effective: "I got waxed today," she told me.

I must have raised an eyebrow.

"Do you want to see?" she asked.

I swallowed, nodded. She was wearing a very short skirt and high heels. She leaned back into the corner of the cab, spread her legs (she had beautiful legs), and pulled her panties to the side with one hand, casting her spell. I stared, transfixed.

"Do you want to touch it? It's really smooth."

I picture myself nodding like an idiot. I leaned forward and ran my fingers along her hairless lips, then soon began to finger her. **At which point we entered a kind of erotic black hole, in which the city not only disappeared but time and space stopped.** It was all gone. I was gone—totally oblivious to everything else but Maggie's freshly waxed pussy.

I'm not sure how long I fingered her like that. It might have been a small but blissful eternity. But suddenly she screamed, and I snapped back to being in the back of a taxi in New York City. I realized that not only had we stopped, but the taxi driver was staring at us over the front seat with a look of transfixed animal desire on his face—probably not unlike the look on my own face.

Mortified, I instantly pulled my fingers out of Maggie and rushed from the taxi, leaving poor Maggie to pay for the ride. She joined me a minute later on the sidewalk, shocked and laughing, and explained to me that the driver had given her his card, telling her she could ride in his cab any time she wanted.

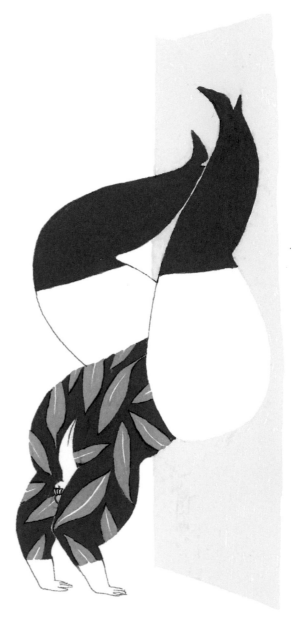

Atieh Sohrabi

Once I was in a car service going to New Jersey from New York City. I was really young, and it was costing me money I didn't have, but it was a remote area and I had no clue how to get there. I was going for an appointment with a therapist who was supposed to be able to help me feel less anxious. I was nervous about the money I was spending on the car service and nervous about the money I was going to spend on the therapist. And also I was running late because we hit traffic. I got so anxious that I had an orgasm in the back seat. That has never happened to me again.

Sometimes you can have a boner and you're not even horny. It's more that you're just comfortable. The morning wood is just that you got to go pee. But you can get a boner just lying on the couch or sitting in a chair—again, not horny, just comfortable. I have been in professional meetings and your mind starts wondering and it starts growing and you gotta think of other things.

I've had moments when someone's been on their period and they say, "No—you don't have to." But this one time I said, "No—let's go for it." **We put down a trash bag, and the blood provided lubrication; I slid in and out.** Then when I stood up, she said, "It looks like you murdered someone!"

I was fully covered in blood. I would only do that with someone I know well.

Once, in the early days, my boyfriend was laid out naked on his back and I was doing whatever combination of things I could come up with—hands and mouth—to deliver him an orgasm. **So I'm crouched down at his crotch, trying some things out, when I realize he's going to come soon.** So I switch to just hand for the last of it, looking back and forth between his face and his boner.

He comes, and time stops.

I watch his face change from bliss to realization and shock to reflexively slamming his eyes shut and trying to turn his face. Through some marvel of physics, the force of ejaculation and the angle of his penis combine to create the perfect projectile arc high over his torso and down, directly between his own eyes. He managed to get his face about two inches to the right before it landed. He absolutely took his own load in his face!

At the time I kept it together and apologized and helped him clean up, a bit mortified. I don't know if he could see the towering laughter in my eyes. But looking back, having seen a bunch of ridiculous hetero porn and having experimentally said okay to a couple face shots, I find it unbelievably hysterical.

We were in high school, late 1990s. Him, two years older. Date at the drive-in theater—I think *Titanic* was playing. Making out in the car, it was my first time kissing with tongue. Gradually I became aware of him saying something…it sounded like, "Immmmmaaacummalloveryou."

"What?" I asked, coming up for air. "What did you say?"

"Immmmmaaacummall-overyou." Half moan, half growl. I still didn't understand. A few seconds went by—maybe a full minute—then it registered: "I'm gonna come all over you."

Our hands were above the waist—above the shoulders, really. Fully clothed (my T-shirt was from dELiA*s). Not even close to third base. Nor second. We were in my dad's 1987 Pontiac Bonneville, and I was pretty sure the soccer mom in the minivan next to us was watching.

But he was gonna come all over me?

DATING & HOOKUPS

SHAINA I once dated a guy who was *much* older than me, and I stayed at his house, and the next morning I realized he had a diamond on his front tooth. Which is totally fine–it was just unexpected because he was really old.

JULIA How drunk were you not to notice a diamond on his front tooth?

SHAINA I wasn't drunk at all! I guess I wasn't paying that much attention to his smile.

Before the internet, there were classifieds. I saw one for a SWF in the *Village Voice* around 1998. The ad said, "You must be into music." And I was into music, so I answered her ad. We went to a diner and had tea. **She looked like someone from the gathering of the Juggalos.** Her shirt said "Bad Religion" with an upside-down cross and she had Manic Panic hair color and looked like she came out of Hot Topic. I thought, *She is definitely too corny.*

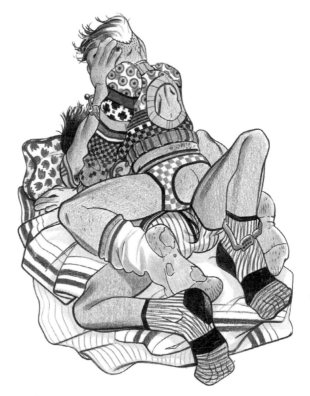

Jeremy Sorese

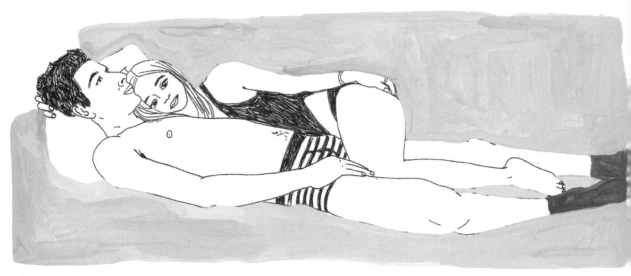

Julia Rothman

Given the era we are in, there's a lot of cultural capital for straight white men to display a kind of empathic, well-versed vocabulary around gender relations and the "woke bae." Of course I've been seduced by that—it's really exciting to me—but every time, I've been shockingly surprised by how it's used as a mode of seduction. I think of this one guy, met him online, had a great conversation, invited me over to read Adrienne Rich poetry. **Immediately afterward, he threw a tantrum because I refused to have unprotected sex with him.**

I have online dated, but it's a waste of time. **I'm more interested in getting to know someone face-to-face and having a real conversation.** Seeing someone's face change and how they speak is all part of the attraction for me. From my experience, with apps I'm meeting an avatar and not a real person. Sometimes people are one-dimensional—especially with Tinder. It's just a way to present oneself. I want to meet in a happenstance way. Most of the relationships I have pursued came after meeting someone in a natural way.

We dated for a year and a half. **She sent me a breakup text.** It sucked. I was like, *Damn, it's over just like that.* After we broke up, I dated a lot, had fun, but nothing lasted. I think it's good. It gave me time to do some soul-searching, getting back to who I am and loving myself. I was so worried about work, was traveling a lot. Shortly after that, she got married. Then she invited me to the wedding, which I thought was a trash-ass move. I politely declined the invitation.

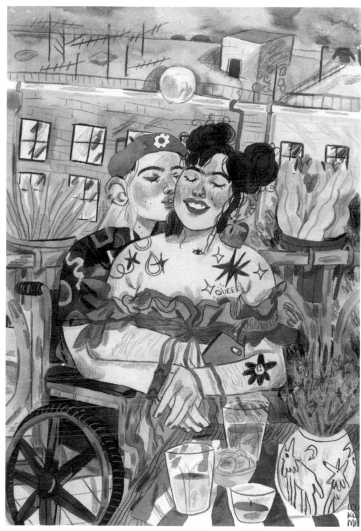

Eleni Koumi

I started dating this guy who was like Prince Charming: he was super-nice with me and my friends, writing me nice messages and being really interested. After two weeks of dating, we had sex at his studio and it was fun—at least for me.

After that, everything changed. He started to act like I didn't matter, like if because I gave him my *tesorito* ("treasure" in Spanish) I gave all my worth and there was no purpose in getting to know me better.

I come from a macho society where if you enjoy yourself, sex, and your body, you get judged and treated like a slut. Luckily, I soon realized it wasn't my fault. I recovered my self-love and told him I didn't want to be with him anymore because his attitude made me feel worthless.

Two months after breaking up, I started dating a new guy. When I gave him my *tesorito,* he started to love me even more. He treated me like I was worth everything because I was myself, and he loved that. Now we are married.

I've done OkCupid, Tinder, Coffee Meets Bagel, Bumble, the League. **I met my boyfriend of six months on OkCupid.**

A lot of times I've gone out for the first time with a woman and it's gone well. **Then the point comes for sex, but no one has a condom and she gets mad at me.** But I wasn't assuming we were going to have sex! We don't even know each other—why would I come with condoms? And then the fact that she doesn't have them either...why is it my responsibility?

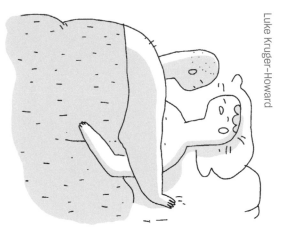

"Say my Twitter handle."

I'm European originally, born and raised in Iceland. The way we look at sex is way more open—way more liberal. **You aren't crucified by your friends and family if you have loads of sex partners.** If you have more than ten sex partners, it's not a bad thing. I remember seeing a movie somewhere, and the main character's friends were judging her for having more than ten sex partners. She was saying, "Oh, my next one has to be my last and the one I marry because I can't have more than ten guys I've slept with."

I think that's a horrible thing—women are just as horny as men! If men can sleep with loads of women, why can't women do the same? I've slept with over sixty guys, and it's a number that I'm really proud of. I'm twenty-nine now, and I started having sex when I was sixteen. I was single for four years and was like, *You know, I'm gonna love myself.*

I don't want to be in a relationship. I still have needs, urges. I still want to have sex. I would sleep around. It sounds really slutty, but I would be pleased.

I met him on Facebook just eight days after my husband died. He was thirty and I was forty-five, and I hadn't been with another man for twenty-three years. When we started texting a couple of weeks later, it got sexy really quickly. He sent me a video of himself jerking off and I was surprised by how much I liked it. Within twenty-four hours, he was on his way to my house so we could have sex.

That day I met him in person, I felt like I had never been more attracted to anyone in my life. And once we started talking, we were having so much fun that we kept forgetting to make out. Once we started really kissing, it turned out that he couldn't get an erection. I think he was hoping for a fast fantasy fuck and accidentally found a friend. I also suspect that he was at a point where he could get it up only with strangers, and that would help to explain why he was pursuing me with such urgency.

Still, meeting him that day was the best, most sexy thing that's ever happened to me. I had never felt so free—had never expressed myself so openly with a man—and that spark of connection when we met was so profound for both of us that we stayed in touch for months after.

EVERY

Underwear Drop

by **PIERA GELARDI**

I don't know if I fell asleep briefly after we had sex, but I was in a haze of groggy confusion as he rushed me to leave his apartment. I was fumbling with the covers in the dark, searching clumsily under the bed for my underwear as he stood over me, impatiently shooing me out. "Go. Go!" he said. I glanced up at him, indignant. Then, conciliatorily, he offered, "I'll mail them to you, okay?" He looked strangely sincere in the moment, but I was dubious. He really, *really* didn't seem like the type to send snail mail.

I remember the door closing. My friend Rhea and I walking down the long staircase in silence: each processing our experience, dazed.

She had told me about the party. "Tuesday we should go to this thing. Cody from Supreme invited me...his friend Ian is house-sitting a siiiick apartment in the East Village. There'll be free booze. It's gonna be really cool."

I was new to the city, from a tiny town in Maine. Hungry for experience, for fun, for big-city life, for excitement. Hungry to no longer be small-town. It sounded like a place to be.

The whole thing was a set-up.

We showed up at the apartment on Tenth Street with our friend Jocelyn, excitedly climbing the stairs to the third-story loft. Inside wasn't a party (*yet,* I thought). In the expansive apartment sat two guys: Rhea's "friend" and his house-sitting skater friend—a lithe, thirty-year-old Peter Pan type with ash-brown long hair and a boyish grin. When they saw there were three of us, there was a commotion: hurried, hushed phone calls I quickly realized were them attempting to find another guy for an even matchup—three girls, three guys. Jocelyn was smart—she saw what was going on and immediately said she had to bounce. I'm smart too, but for whatever reason I stayed.

What happened next I imagine in the style of one of those made-for-TV special scenes where everything is sped up, and the footage includes trails or other hallucinatory effects to show the depraved nature of what's happening. There was free booze as promised, drugs were trotted out, and we paired off. I remember a deep, drug-fueled conversation with Ian on the patio, a canopy of trees, the night sky. For a moment, it all seemed dreamy. Then things inevitably transitioned into what the night was designed for, and an intense, acrobatic fuck fest ensued.

Rhea and I stepped down the last step of the long staircase, through the door, and out onto an empty Twelfth Street in the wee hours. We heard the door click behind us and turned to each other, filled with experiences to dish.

Then all of a sudden I heard him calling my name.

Everything became slow motion, the streetlights glimmered, my head tilted up to behold him silhouetted in the open door of the balcony above. Something white fluttered down toward me through the night. My heart swelled—was it a love note? His number?

I still don't know how I possibly thought this might be a romantic moment, my own Romeo and Juliet scene. But I honestly did.

And then the object came into focus and my panties hit the pavement. The end of romance.

Just kidding. I wish the misadventure had ended there.

Improbably, the next morning I woke up convinced that this was a relationship with potential. I sat in my kitchen on Avenue C, surrounded by my roommates, who helped me write Ian a letter. I wrote it in rainbow markers, a different color for each line, each line a funny excuse for why I had stopped by Ian's apartment again:

I love tennis and thought you might want to play doubles.

I baked cookies and know how you love snickerdoodles.

I think I left my Atari at your apartment.

The list went on. Then I crossed everything out and wrote *Call me?* at the bottom. I went by the Twelfth Street apartment and left the note on the door.

Of course, he never called.

I think back to this time in my life often, slightly baffled by my sex life.

My hunger for experience drove me at this age. I painted and drew and made videos. I was never without my camera in hand, exploring, documenting. I scoured the *New York Times* and *Time Out* for interesting happenings and was out every night: a poetry reading, a jazz club, a Laurie Anderson art opening, the Mermaid Parade, Wigstock, dancing to techno at Twilo. I hosted dinner parties. I was sparkly, fun, and full of love to give. I was the type of person who sent snail mail. Yet I was constantly in these hazy one-night-stand situations where I thought a person who didn't care about me in the slightest was *the one.*

Years later, I ran into the long-haired housesitter at a party. He smiled sheepishly as he approached. I hated to admit it, but I still thought he was sexy. We exchanged small talk, then he paused and told me, "You know, I still have that note you left me back in the day. It's the coolest thing anyone's ever made for me."

WHAT I LIKE

JULIA Remember when that crowd of women were telling us about the soaps they use on their vaginas before they have sex?

SHAINA Yeah. Have you tried any of them out?

JULIA Not yet.

Before sex, you take a nice warm bath. You get yourself all ready. Let me tell you my secret: I use Dr. Bronner's peppermint soap on my coochie. That makes it feel tingly and fresh. Like when you chew gum and you drink water and it feels all fresh? That's how it makes your coochie feel.

First serious girlfriend introduced me to a lot of different sensations I wasn't even aware turned me on. **One occasion we were making out and she stuck her tongue as far down my ear as she could.** I thought to myself, *What the hell is this girl doing?* But I didn't want to ruin the mood, so I pretended to like it. She kept doing it whenever we made out and had sex. I don't know when it happened, but eventually I didn't have to pretend anymore—even got to the point where I would ask her for an "ear job"!

I like wearing clothes and someone telling me to take them off: "Hey, take your panties off and spread your legs." I like them to boss me around a little bit. Not a whole bunch of kinky shit —I'm not a submissive person—but you gotta tell me that you want the pussy. And you have to be ready to eat vagina, because that's what I like. You gotta be able to work your tongue. **I want all the swirls up and down.** If he slips to my booty, that's a good thing.

My girlfriend and I are working on me being eaten out more. **It's hard for me to be vulnerable.**

We were in bed one night and we were messing around, and my husband said to me, "You have a lovely body." After being with someone for thirteen years, it was a very sweet and profoundly erotic thing for him to say. **Sometimes it's the little things.**

I like my pussy bald. **No hair.** I put coconut oil on my coochie. And it feels all good and soft and moist.

As far as relationships, I'm
trans-romantic. On a day-
to-day basis I find all
bodies hot, but I like to date
people who are going through
the experience of being
trans, like me. Whether
medically or not. Someone
who is on that spectrum.

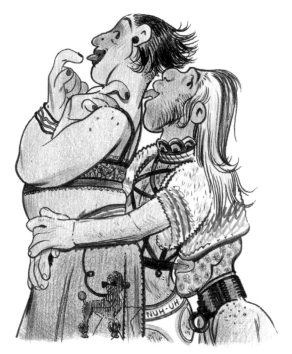

Jeremy Sorese

I have a dirty mouth. I've always liked to talk in bed, in a whisper in the car or a low mumble. I remember the first time I carefully instructed a lover to give me a blow job. I don't know where this intense, badass, bad-boy voice came from, but it came quite naturally. Step by step.

I remember I had a blue strap-on cock from a previous relationship. I was wearing it. Cock pulled out of the underpants for her to hold. She stroked it. The harness was leather and had shiny silver sparkles. She was on her knees, a gorgeous femme with dark curly hair. I was sitting on the side of her bed. She licked and swallowed it and stroked according to my instructions. The cock was veiny and floppy, but hard. When I wear a cock, it's always an extension of me and my identity when I have sex. That never seemed confusing to me. Base of the cock pushed on me and it felt good against my parts. I was getting off. She was wet and eager to please. I love telling her what to do. Topping. Years later, she told a friend it was the best sex she'd ever had. Eventually we fucked. There were a lot of breathy claims and ultimatums. We both came. Very butch/femme. Very fun. Obviously, I never forgot. Dirty and special.

I love nipples and the small of the back. And also just the vagina-butthole combo—it is so perfect. I don't think you can say you're eating pussy if you're not eating her ass at some point. I always think those two things go hand in hand. And I like belly buttons. And nice hair.

One time I got stoned and my girlfriend at the time gave me head, and **I felt like I saw a new color.**

Sometimes when my wife gets angry at me and yells at me to do stuff, I get a boner. **I guess it's some dominant shit where even if she tells me to do the dishes, I get turned on.** It's strange.

I love group sex because there's hands everywhere. I would have my tongue in someone and then my hands would be on different people. **I've had one woman sitting on my face and another riding me.** Just the intermingling of bodies—it's like Twister! I love it. It's wild.

I like his dad bod. The squishiness. **It's uncomfortable when someone is hard.**

I look for good dick. It has to be nice, firm, veins. **Veins turn me on.** I can feel it when it's going in and out of my pussy. Curved, if possible; that's easier to hit the G-spot.

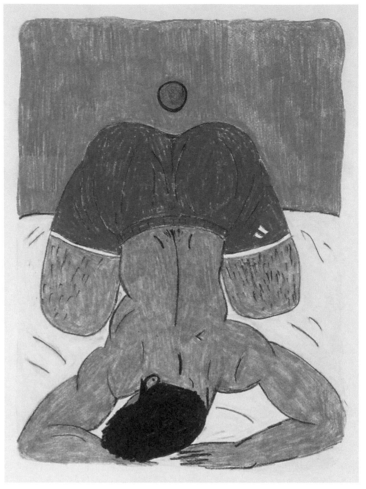

Soufiane Ababri

I'm thirty-seven. My girl is fifty-two years old. **When we first started having sex I'd just pound away, but it didn't really do much for her.** She doesn't come through penetration. So I figured out that if I take my penis and bang it against her clitoris, she'll come. The first time I tried it, she came like fifteen times. Most people are saying, *Oh, you gotta pound them.* Not true.

I'm thirty-one, been having sex since I was seventeen, and don't even know how many partners I've had. But my current boyfriend was the first person ever to make me squirt. I'm one of the lucky ones who can have orgasms from just penis in vagina; I don't need to manipulate my clitoris to have an orgasm. It's really good when I have one. **I can feel my whole body tensing up and my eyes roll back in my head—I'm shaking.** And I'll have back-to-back orgasms. It's ridiculous.

For some reason or another, I love giving oral sex to my partner. It just really turns me on and makes me so wet. And whenever I get really worked up, I can really go to town. One time I was doing it and my boyfriend cried from how good it felt—I made him cry!

To prepare, I Nair. **You gotta keep it tight.**

I like older women because they tend to know sexually what they need better. **That's not to degrade younger women.** It's just that older women—thirty-five and up—tend to take you and say, *Look we're both gonna get off, but I need you to do this first, and I need you to be here.* That communication is just key. Not everyone does that—particularly younger women, from my experience.

We were sitting on my bed watching a movie together, side by side. She was my Tinder match, but she knew it was my first time with a girl. The movie had barely started and you could feel the sexy tension in the air. Suddenly our fingers touched, sending a wave of electricity all over my body. A while later, she took my hand into hers and slowly moved her thumb over the palm of my hand. I stroked her hand back and she pulled my arm over her lap. I turned my head a bit, she looked at me, we kissed. Softly at first. I held her face and she held my waist. I slowly moved my hands downward and touched her breast, as if accidentally. Her body shook slightly and she held me tightly. She put her hand on my inner thigh and I took off her top. I kissed her nipples while she stroked me between my legs. I was super-wet.

She slid one finger inside me and I moaned—I couldn't hold it in. I stopped doing anything and just focused on what her finger was doing to me. She made me come so easily, like no man had ever done. She smiled at me, proud of what she'd done, but with a look on her face that said *I do it all the time—get used to it.*

Then it was my turn to please her. I kissed her lips, then her nipples and stomach. She was shaking with pleasure. I held her thighs apart and kissed her, then slid a finger inside her, then two. She tasted warm and sexy. I was so horny just to see how wet she was. She came. After that, we didn't just lie in bed like I used to with guys. She started kissing me again, her red curls between my thighs. I didn't think I could, but I came again. Then I made her come again. At some point we got tired and spooned to sleep for a while.

I woke up with her hand between my legs. I was still wet from the night before, and still horny. We kissed and rolled on my bed—half-horny and half-lazy, having just woken up. We had sex for a long while, then I had to go. I didn't want to, but I had a plane to catch.

That was more than a year ago. I never saw her again, but I think of her all the time when I touch myself, hoping that I will someday have another experience as delicious as she was.

She was older than me. I was twenty-eight at the time. She was forty-nine. I met her at a bar and she just kind of hooked onto me and didn't let me go, and it made me feel really like *It's going down tonight.* I wanted her to come back to my place because she was from out of town, but she wasn't comfortable. So we just got in her car and went somewhere. She had this very small Toyota, and I was like *I'm gonna make it work.* I really wanted it to happen.

At the end of the day, it was really good. I never knew sex in a car would be that good. I wasn't prepared for what she taught me. It wasn't just that she was an older woman. She really put it on me. One example is that in this very small car, the seats were all the way leaned back and her face was against her back window, basically, and I'm behind her, doggy-style. And I don't know how it happened, but she stopped and flipped me over—maybe because I was unbalanced—and she was kind of like, *It's my turn.* I was like, *Okay, this is fun.* I'm a big guy, and she just flips me over and starts riding me. And I'm like, *How in the hell did this happen?* I don't know, but I'm going with it. I'm just taken.

From the very beginning, she was like, *Tonight you're mine—and you don't have a choice.* And I'm like, *I'm okay with that.* It opened up a fire in me I didn't know I had. I like a woman being very aggressive. I like whips, chains, and stuff. But for a woman to say what she wants, how she wants it, leave no gray area—that is critical. Particularly in today's climate, when you never want to step over that boundary. She was just like, *This is what I want.* That's dope to me.

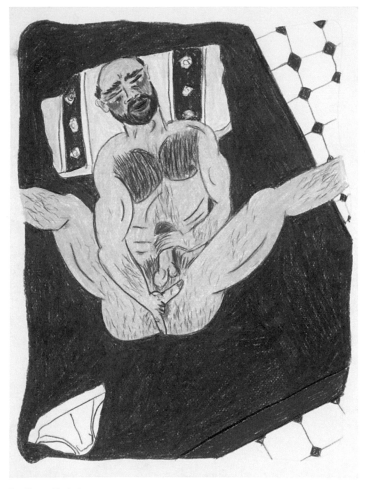

Soufiane Ababri

My favorite thing is alternating between vaginal and oral sex. **If your partner is on all fours, you can service them both ways.**

We'd both had previous partners and had known each other for only a few months. The chemistry was palpable and persistent. He proposed, suddenly. I accepted. We knew sex before, but not with each other. We knew we didn't want our commitment to be about our bodies. **We decided to remain celibate until we got married.**

It was painful, but we were resolute: this time, this relationship, would be different.

On our wedding night, we stalled. We opened presents. He slowly removed ninety-six bobby pins from my updo. Slowly we went upstairs. Casual, like nothing was about to happen.

When he finally entered me, tears streamed down my face from bliss and peace and lack of shame. I cried the entire time from an ecstasy wrapped in peace.

Seventeen years later, he makes me climax in an instant. Vaginal orgasms are his regular gift to me—in addition to five beautiful babies.

Some things are worth the wait.

I'm a PG slut—I love kissing everyone. But that's about it. I kiss people way more than the average human; it's like my handshake. In a consensual way, of course!

I've tried anal a few times, but I'm not really into it. **It's next door to one of the greatest places on Earth.**

I like it when a guy bites my lips—my vaginal lips—and bites the clit! That's good head.

I look at porn to see women squirt. And then I had a girl who was a squirter and it blew my mind. It was so different. To see a woman have multiple orgasms and then release that. It was a really good experience.

I took a trip to Sweden and I had some girl fuck me with a dildo and it was cool.

I like older women. They want a guy who's young and has energy and isn't boring. And I like the wisdom. **Women are naturally more mature than men, so you're adding even more years to it.** I feel so bad for guys who have to look at teenage porn. It's usually nineteen-year-olds who are legal, but dressing like fifteen-year-olds. I click on the MILF stuff.

I was recently with a woman who was fifty years old—more than a decade older than me. **It was great because I knew she couldn't have kids, and I didn't want to have kids, so we just had fun.** At this age, and as New Yorkers, whether you want kids comes up so much faster. I don't want to lead someone on. Some people within four, six weeks, their gears start turning for the picket fence and the dog and the kids. Before you even talk about it, you can see it in people's reactions—how they view the kid in the stroller coming toward you. Do they stop to pet dogs or say hi to the baby?

John Cuneo

An orgasm for me is an eruption. It's something to experience from head to toe. And if I can't get engaged enough with my partner to get her to have an orgasm, it's kind of, *Eh*. I want to be able to give an orgasm as well as get one. **Sometimes it's just the buildup of the entire day—a text, a little note.** I've sent pictures. What I have enjoyed sending in the past, it wasn't just a regular old picture, but it left something to the imagination. I was covered up. Naughty, without being too much.

It's gotta be the right mood, the right moment. A lot of guys are done in five, six minutes: *bam bam bam* and they're done. **You gotta slow them down, ease them into it.** A lot of times it's not what you say, it's how you say it. You push them back, slow it down, and just guide their hands. A man wants to just grope. I say, *Smooth me, caress me, hold me a moment.* And then at the end he will see the reward is better than the *bam bam bam.* He's happy, you're happy.

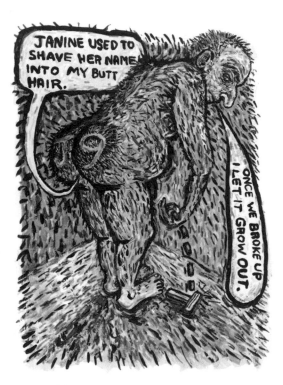

Dave Zackin

I always cringe a little when I hear someone say something like *Sex, being a universal human desire...* or *The most basic human need, sex.* Sex has always felt like something I was supposed to go along with and eventually start to enjoy. After five years of having sex occasionally, I have realized that it was all the weird messaging I received around sex that made it so problematic for me. That I had to look good doing it, and make sure my partner's needs were always being met, that I was groomed and hairless and ready, that I was chill and fun and "sexy."

For the first time ever, with my current partner I am enjoying sexual interactions—largely because we are doing what is fun for *us,* but might not be what is most typically represented as what sex between a cis man and a cis woman looks like. Once when I told my friend about what we were doing, she quipped, "But you're not really having sex, then, are you?" We need to overcome the notion that P-V penetration is some finish line or goal that all cis man /cis woman pairings are aspiring to perfect. There are ways to enjoy each other's bodies that don't follow the poses that all rom-com sex scenes look like.

I'm really excited to be at the beginning of enjoying my sex life, even though it took longer than I wanted to get here, and even though it's still awkward and unsatisfying sometimes. There's something fun about feeling like we are rewriting the sexual playbook.

It was between me and my stepbrother. **He was fresh out of the shower and I saw him naked and got a great view of his penis.** I knew I wanted him inside me at that moment so I went to my room, lay naked on the bed, and called him in. It only took about ten seconds for us to start touching each other, and things got sexually physical. The idea of us being somewhat related and having sex really turned me on, which gave me multiple orgasms.

Once we finished, we both went about our day as if nothing happened. We do this about once or twice a week.

I've gotten a dick pic before. He was a large man—some guy I met on Craigslist. I was looking through the ads and I picked him. I asked him for it. **And I wanted to see it again and again, so I'd request it again and again from him.** His dick was at least eight or nine inches, and it wasn't small around either.

We'd meet up and have sex. The first time, it was a lot of fun. But after that he got more and more rough. I'm a small person and he was not a small person, so I started to not enjoy it.

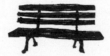

Sex in Parks

by REN KHODZHAYEV

The first time I had sex in a park, it wasn't sex per se. Viviana and I met on Tinder—she was married but open, very smart, with a filthy mind. However, after weeks of dirty talk it was all still imaginary. So I proposed we meet in Fort Greene Park, telling her, *Come and look for me, but if you find me, you're not allowed to speak. Walk up and kiss me like you've missed me for a long time.*

A maxim that everyone knows by now is that the Tinder self rarely shows up IRL. I didn't know how tall Viv was or what she looked like when she smiled—I still hadn't even heard her voice—yet I found myself on a park bench, failing to concentrate on my book, chain-smoking with shaking hands, scanning the path in both directions, unsure whether she would show up. When she did, she mouthed *Hello* and folded herself into

my arms. I smelled her neck and her hair, and she rubbed her face against my chest, and then we kissed. She sucked on my tongue and bit my lip; then she put her hand up my shirt and ran her fingernails down my back. We were two strangers meeting for the first time, and what got me off the most was that to the rest of the world, we looked like two people in love.

The second time I had sex in a park was with Kim. She texted me one night, but I'd already had sex that day and, even worse, I didn't remember who Kim was—we'd never met in real life. *We met on an app,* she reminded me, and I said, *Thanks Kim, but I'm all fucked out.* She replied, *I bet I could make you come again.*

We met at midnight, again in Fort Greene Park, and sat on a bench for the three minutes it took her to decide I wasn't a rapist. Then we went to the tennis courts. At first we fucked up against the fence, but the rattling of the chain links made me nervous, so we got down on the ground. The sex was fun because, despite the late hour, I could sense people watching us, but it didn't actually feel very pleasant. On top of me, Kim seemed a bit histrionic, as if she were acting out a role rather than enjoying herself. At one point she reached down to make sure I'd really put a condom on; that hurt my feelings a little bit, but what could I say? We were strangers.

Our goodbye was about as warm as the rest of it, and I didn't really expect to see her again, but when she booty-called me a few weeks later, I came. And I kept going until Kim decided that she liked me.

I couldn't submit to a relationship with Kim, because I didn't want to give up the high I was getting from my Tinder connections. However, as soon as Kim and I broke up, the high stopped working. I continued hooking up with strangers—a bartender in Lefferts, a film editor in Bushwick, girls whose names I don't remember—and each of those encounters made me feel worse than the one before. Still, I couldn't stop myself. I talked about it in therapy and even went to 12-step meetings for sex addicts, all in the hopes of trying to bring this behavior under control. However, as my AA sponsor pointed out to me, these things weren't actually in my control and, in his experience, I wouldn't stop until I was ready—whatever *that* meant.

In the following months I moved to Europe and tried to date "normally," but then I matched with Catherine. She was a writer with a pretty romantic sensibility, and she told me that her fantasy was to be *taken* by a stranger in the woods. At night the parks in our city are dark and gloomy, and a thunderstorm was rolling in as I headed to meet her. Since I was new in town, I got lost and found myself stumbling around the dark, dense trees, cell phone in hand, texting *where r u?* By the time I found her, Catherine had relocated to a playground. Sitting on a wooden

replica of Aladdin's carpet, she seemed calm and collected, while I was in no position to *take* anyone. We tried nonetheless, but all we did was act out an approximation of desire. Catherine applied her skills with a determined efficiency—later, I learned that she'd spent a year working in a brothel as research for a book—while I spent half the time wondering: *Is that broken glass digging into my back?*

I did not succeed in *taking* Catherine, and afterward she returned none of my calls. Before we parted she told me about her other books, her child, her long-term partner. Despite myself I wanted a connection with her, while she wanted me only for a specific function. Her radio silence hurt, and I kept trying to text her, attempting to undo my failure. But trying to undo this one was like trying to push an amputated finger back onto its bloody stump and, in a state of post-traumatic shock, believing it will stick.

Although she was unavailable, Catherine had given me a glimpse of what I really desired—connection—and this led me to a new Tinder bottom. Again I reached out to my recovery friends. We did some "step work" around it, and then I deleted my profile, deleted all the apps, called it quits.

Unfortunately, addiction isn't cured by quitting. Before long, I was digging up old numbers I had stored in my phone.

Franzi was the first woman I matched with after I moved to Europe; she opened our conversation by asking to get fucked in the ass. Though it was a fun and depraved beginning, I began to despise myself after seeing her. While she enjoyed anal sex as a sort of antidepressant, I was starting to feel ashamed of stranger-fucking, beginning to sense that it was draining my self-esteem. But when it sunk in that Catherine would never talk to me again, my self-esteem was so low that I figured it wouldn't matter if I called Franzi again. I figured things couldn't get any worse.

And so, on a gray winter afternoon, I found myself fucking Franzi from behind while she ground her pubis against an industrial-size vibrator, practically yelling at me to fuck her harder. That's when I noticed there were splatters of shit all over me. From where I was, I could see myself in the mirror—sweaty and vacant, covered in shit, pounding into a woman I felt nothing for, a woman clearly as desensitized as I was. I figured it was easier to keep going than to stop, but in doing so I tried not to touch her. Afterward I went straight to the bathroom, and as I sat in her tub hosing myself off, Franzi came in and asked me to piss in her mouth.

But let me end this story back where it began, in another park with another stranger. This time it was with an Eastern European academic, on the first nice day of spring, alongside a stream, watching the ducks swim past. While our conversation started out normally, one topic led to another, and the academic began telling me how she can make herself come simply by squeezing her pussy. Then we began making out, and lying there with our limbs intertwined we looked like two lovers simply holding each other in the grass; in reality the academic had her crotch pressed against me and I was pulling her hair and sticking my fingers in her mouth, and she was spasming orgasms, over and over, on my leg.

It didn't get me off at all.

When I first got on Tinder, I came up with an analogy to describe what I was looking for. Picture an x-y graph, where y signifies the ultimate fuck-a-stranger fantasy and x represents time. Y was highest when $x=0$, because the more time I spent with a stranger, the more I got to know them. With time, their humanity came into focus and feelings came into play—and back then I didn't want any feelings.

My friend Rebecca's theory is that I was trying to seduce every woman I came across because I didn't get enough love from my mother. My theory is that after my last relationship, which left me feeling undesirable and sexually inept, I needed to know that I was still fuckable. Whereas the two theories have different underlying moti-

vations, they essentially amount to the same thing: I was trying to fuck my way to self-worth. A fool's errand, as I ultimately discovered, because on the actual, existential plane my fantasy quickly turned into a high, and then just an escape from self—the new, lower self I became after each encounter.

During this slide down the y-axis, I've had women, postcoitally or even mid-sex, ask me what my name was. The first time I thought it was funny, but it was a joke that worked only once. These days I pray they have since forgotten my name—as I've forgotten most of theirs—and that if we do meet again, we can do so anew. This time, however, it will be to *connect* as people, not just as a pile of disembodied parts—or, more aptly, not like strangers on a sinking ship, clinging to the nearest bit of warmth, senselessly hoping to *escape* what looms beneath the surface.

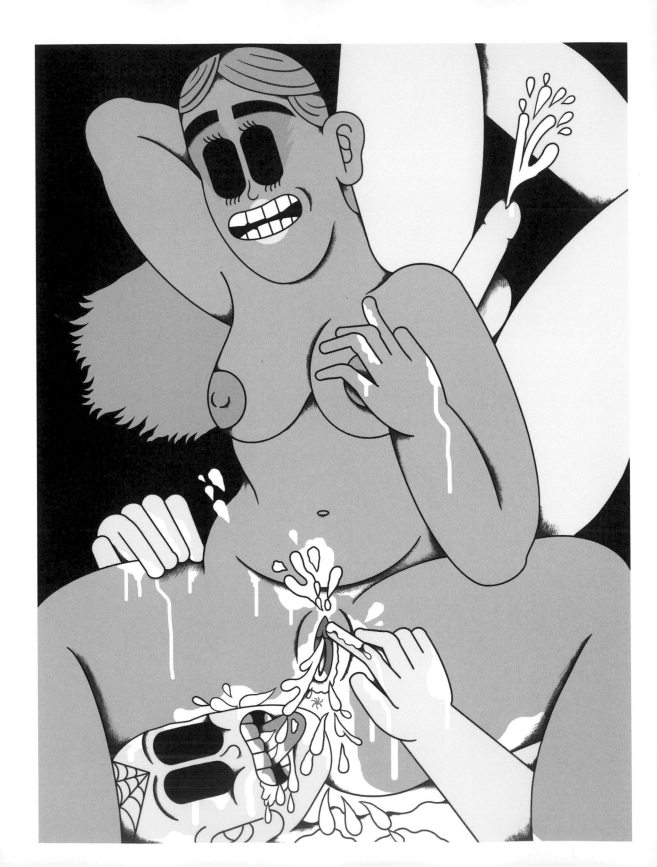

LOCATION, LOCATION, LOCATION

John F. Malta

JULIA Have you made out with anyone in a taxi?

SHAINA Uh, yeah—I'm from New York.

JULIA Yeah, I guess it's a rite of passage for all New Yorkers.

I used to have sex in my car. **It was a tiny car.** We would roll the seats to the front and get in the back seat. The windows would fog up. The whole car would move. It always hurt my knees.

I dated this guy and he wore a suit every day, and he was so buttoned-up and uptight. He brought me to his office one time and took me on a tour. And then all of a sudden he put me on his desk and ate me out, and then he turned me around—on his desk—and started doing me. He also loved to spank me, and he'd make me crawl on the floor and pull my hair. It wasn't mean—it was hot.

I had sex outside. In the park. It was wild. Late night. Beautiful night. **We wanted something fun and experimental.** Missionary, from the back, doggy-style, I rolled a couple times. It was nice. I'm an adventurous person, so I like taking risks.

We were driving his dad to the airport after a track meet. His grandmother was driving a big SUV, his fifteen- and three-year-old sisters were in the middle row of seats, and we were in the very back. He started fingering me, and I ended up giving him a blow job right there in the back of the car, with four of his family members oblivious to it. We were seventeen.

The craziest place I ever had sex was the beach. I had gone to Myrtle Beach with my ex-girlfriend, and we were feeling amorous. It was broad daylight. My family was sitting there on the sand. **We were in the ocean, so nobody could see anything.** It's really buoyant because you float. It was kind of a hot turn-on, because I was saying *Fuck you* to my parents but they didn't know.

Some places I've had sex: on the BART train, in a restroom at a bar, on Market Street in the middle of the street, at a club, in the milk freezer of a supermarket, in the bathroom of a coffee shop I worked at, on a lifeguard stand at Rockaway Beach. **I'm a total whore.**

I'm a retired police officer, and yes I got a blow job in a police car.

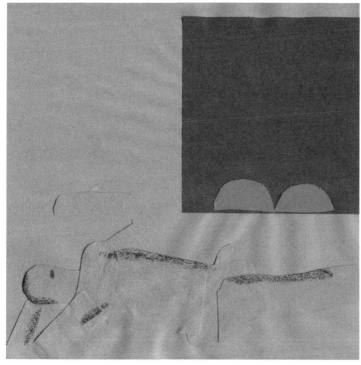

Josh Cochran

I was in South Africa. I went wine tasting, and I met this guy. I was getting drunk, and we started making out. We decided to move away from the group and it was getting late, with everyone heading off to sleep. **So he and I are up against this tree making out, and it was so hot.** Then he got down on his knees, took off my panties, put my legs over his shoulders, and ate me out, with my back up against the tree. I was bugging. I was moaning so loud!

The next day everybody was like, *Did you hear those people having sex last night? They were so loud!* And I was like, *That's crazy—I was asleep, I didn't hear anything.* But "those people" were us!

Back in high school I was a stud. I had a full head of hair. I used to get a lot of girls. This one girl I was dating, we were hot and heavy for one another. We were at a Cumberland Farms convenience store and she didn't want to do it in the car, but there was a little alcove where we could climb on top of the roof. She said, "Come on, let's go."

So we climbed on top of the Cumberland Farms and made love up there. I went back inside afterward to buy a pack of cigarettes, and people started applauding me. **Turns out we were on top of the skylight.**

I saw this cute guy from my bio class drinking a beer at a frat party. It was late—probably around 2 a.m.—and he'd had a little too much to drink, but so had I. He kinda recognized me. Then he told me how nice it would be if I could suck his cock, and that nobody would see me because we were behind the bar. I thought maybe he would like me if I did it. I kissed him on the cheek. He pushed my head down hard with one hand and unzipped his jeans. I sucked it, trying to make sure my lips were wet and tucked over my teeth. He came in my mouth, and I swallowed. **Then he zipped his jeans and walked away.**

I'm from Chicago, and I've had sex in a little courtyard on the bench by the Channel 5 news building. It was her idea, so I was all for it. I said, "Okay—let's go!"

Her little brother and his girl-friend were there. They weren't watching, but they were close by. She lifted her skirt and sat on my lap.

INFIDELITY

SHAINA I cheated on someone once and immediately regretted it.

JULIA I've cheated and been cheated on. It's never worth it.

SHAINA You didn't like being cheated on?

JULIA [Eye roll]

We met in Houston; I was driving cross-country. We were both friends of friends who happened to be invited out on the same night. We couldn't get enough of each other and talked until 4 a.m. The next day I was off. This was back when people wrote letters to each other. In my first letter, I told her I regretted not kissing her. She told me she was thinking of me obsessively. We wrote two, three—sometimes five letters a day.

A month later, she showed up at my door and said she was tired of writing letters.

In my experience to that point, sex had been fun but often awkward and rushed—never totally satisfying. Sex was mainly something that happened in the dark. There was nothing awkward about R: she liked the lights on and the windows open. Within ten minutes of arriving at my door, she was naked in the bedroom. She was the first woman who told me what she wanted, and the first one who asked me what I wanted. She saw her body as an instrument that needed to be played. We were both twenty-three and grieving people in our lives who had died tragically, and our bodies offered escape. There was a poetry to the days, which began and ended in a fever of sex. We lived inside each other for that summer. She was competitively orgasmic and wanted to be touched under a blanket in Central Park, in a quiet nook at the Met, or at dinner in a nice restaurant. She wanted me to watch her orgasm and she wanted to push my boundaries and watch me react.

Fevers break, though, reality sets in, and after a few months she was back to her life and I mine. Letters were not enough anymore. The everyday intruded. Marriages and kids and families followed for both of us, and we lost touch. I thought about her for years. She was the one who would intrude in my dreams.

A few years ago at a wedding, she was there. We greeted each other politely, exchanging pleasantries while silently dealing with the sudden aging of the people we hold in our memories. Late into the evening, she caught me looking at her across the room. She nodded me to the door. We escaped, found a room, and fucked with a capital F. It felt as if time had opened up a new thread, and in that moment it was possible to imagine a very different life, one spent together. She cried—happy tears, I think. I felt as if my heart was bursting, but it was too late. **We had just betrayed the people we loved. We dressed and returned to the party. Life was waiting.**

I am having an affair. We make out at Penn Station a lot. People come up to us and say they have never seen that much public display of affection. We are both married. I created a secret life. Every time we get to see each other, I get butterflies, and it's been going on for well over a year—that says something.

We work at an ad agency that has reunions. I met her at one of those two years ago and we stayed in touch, had lunch a few times, then found out about day rates at hotels.

I sometimes think about whether we could be together. But she has kids of her own who are teenagers. I've been married thirty-six years. I met my wife in my mid-twenties and we have two grown boys. I hope I can keep this secret life a secret for a long time, and that we both have our other lives. When you're with the same person for forty years or so, your relationship isn't quite as romantic or sexual, and you still need that. Somehow we figured this out, and we seem to be pretty happy.

I think we are in love. We talk all the time. We text all the time. We say good morning and good night every day. I have never had sex like this before. It makes you think about why people write love songs and make dumb romance movies. I never used to talk when I had sex. Now I can't stop telling her how much I love fucking her. Now I realize why everyone likes sex so much.

I have thought about leaving my wife, but I still love her. You get older and you don't really want to do that to somebody. We share a bed, but we don't have sex. She originally started it by telling me she wasn't interested in sex anymore. But then recently she's been asking, "When are we going to have sex?" It's so complicated!

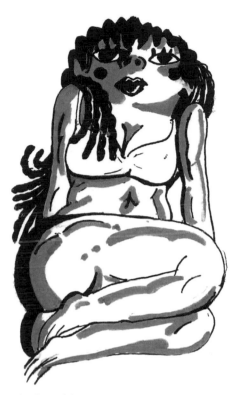

Branche Coverdale

I knew this guy was married, and the only reason I wanted him in the first place was because someone I hate wanted him too—petty, I know! But then when the flirting started, it was electric—he gave me such a rush—but nothing happened because I had to take a friend home. Longing looks were exchanged.

A year later, I saw him again at a party. He was buzzed and so was I, and he just locked in on me. I kept trying to say no, but all the dirty things he discreetly whispered in my ear made me wetter than wet. Finally I couldn't take it anymore; we left the building and had rough and desperate sex in an alleyway.

A few days later he was at another party, this time with his wife. I was there but standing far away, and he kept walking past me and touching me, rubbing himself on me while passing, and I couldn't help myself: we had sex again and again after that. I felt horrible only after the first time.

She gave me a Batman T-shirt for my birthday and pressed her whole body against me. I became obsessed with the desire to understand if this was a Mexican cultural thing or an expression of interest. It sat in the back of my mind and invaded my thoughts during meetings.

I suppressed the thought because I am the nice guy with two kids and a sensible wife. I am successful, dependable, reliable, and not impulsive. I have a great job and good career. However, I cannot get the *What did that mean?* thought out of my head.

One day we had a family barbecue with beer, which led into late-night wine. She complained that her father said she was fat. My wife and I said he was wrong. Then my wife went to bed.

I said her dad was wrong and she was tiny, and she should stand up and compare herself to me. We stood back to back, and I felt her lace her fingers through mine. We turned, and I could see drunken desire in her eyes.

I smiled and leaned in. She kissed me and I was surprised by the size and thickness of her tongue. I turned her around and kissed her neck. She turned and grinded on my thick thighs. I turned her away from me and kissed her neck again. This time I slipped my hand down inside her jeans, then her panties, and stroked her clitoris. She exploded and spun around, dropping to her knees. She wrestled with my belt. I felt exhilaration and numbness. I instinctively undid my belt. She reached into my trousers and then my boxers and released my penis. I felt fear, guilt, lust, and power. I resisted for a second and then surrendered.

She slid my hard penis into her mouth. Her tongue was thick and sensual. She slid her head back and forth, taking me deeper and deeper, but I still felt numb and removed from the situation. She grabbed my penis and started masturbating it into her mouth. I desperately wanted to come and fill her mouth. I wanted to give her pleasure and picked her up, taking off her jeans and underwear. I guided her to the sofa and looked at her deeply. She tasted of apples or apple-flavored sweets.

I slid inside and made love, then forgot myself and put her legs over my shoulders. I pushed deep inside repeatedly until I came. I felt guilty and satisfied.

We hurriedly got dressed, and she asked me not to tell my wife. That was the first and last happy moment. I lost the next four years to depression.

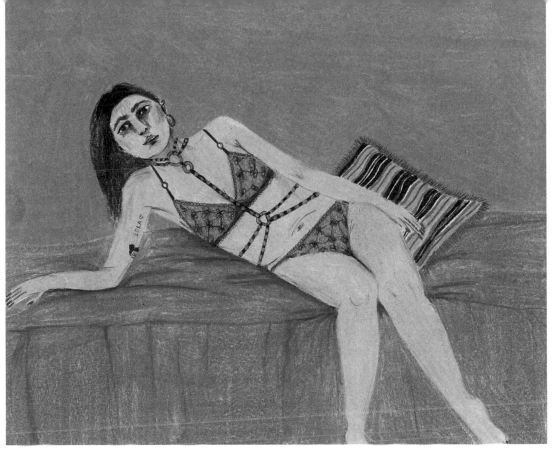

Adriana Lozano

In high school, I had a best friend, Rosa. I would go to her house all the time. I was just coming out of the closet. **I came out to my parents, and my dad kicked me out.** Rosa's parents took me in. I lived there for six months or maybe even a year; it was a while. I was really close with her mom and dad. They would lend me their car, and they fed me.

Fast-forward ten years or so: I'm twenty-eight. I had this thing where I was cruising rest areas. I would go and hook up with guys. We would meet, then go somewhere. One night I went to a rest area and saw Rosa's dad; I was walking up to the rest area and he was walking away. I stopped him and said, "Hey, how's it going?" He was a pretty good-looking man—a DILF for sure. I was super-excited, and we went back to their house. I kept trying to put the moves on him, but nothing happened. I was disappointed. He kept saying, "Oh, I just stopped to take a piss," pretending he wasn't cruising the rest area too. But why else would he be there? His house was like a mile away.

Fast-forward again and we're at our good friend's wedding. Rosa was there with her parents, and it was a whole night of drinking and dancing. It was super-fun, but then the night came to an end and everyone wound up going to a hotel. I decided not to go, and Rosa's parents offered me a ride home. I ended up going back to their house, where Rosa's mom passed out and her dad put the moves on me—*finally*.

That started a two-year-long affair. It wasn't all the time, but every few months we would hook up. It was pretty passionate. Nobody ever found out. I'm still really good friends with them today.

Ohni Lisle

My wife suffers from depression. **Her sex drive was always low, but in the last few years it's been below zero.** She gets mad at me if I even suggest sex. She's also anti-masturbation. I love her and my family, but the physical loneliness wears on me; over time, it can feel excruciating.

It's worse to sleep next to someone you love but who no longer wants to be touched than to sleep alone. After about two years of celibacy, I found myself checking out massage parlors. I had never done anything like that before—never cheated— but I felt overwhelmed by the need for touch. Massage parlors offering a wide range of sexual services are everywhere in New York—easy to find if you know

what to look for. I wasn't going to go to a brothel (too scary). Some massage parlors are scary and scream of sexual slavery; I ran from those. But I've found many that are well run, clean, and dare I say *professional*. They are often run by entrepreneurial women who know we're sad guys looking to get off and escape our lives for a bit. The women are often happy to help in exchange for some cash.

There's a place I go regularly now. It's like therapy: I talk to my gal about my life, and she hers. Often we talk about cooking. We laugh a lot. I find myself feeling totally open in this place— unashamed of my belly. These women have seen everything. The first thing they do is wash

me like a baby, scrubbing every nook and cranny. They wear big rubber rain boots as they pour warm water over you. I like the massage as much as the hand job that comes afterward.

Civilians could learn a thing or two from these women. These aren't just hand jobs—they're hand jobs that make you see God. My gal gets naked for me and lets me touch her boobs while she gets me off. She asks me if I am thinking of my wife. I used to, but now my mind is mainly empty. I'm at peace. I just accept that this is my life. A bit sad and not what I expected it to be, but enough to get me through the day.

As Told To

WHAT YOU MIGHT SEE AT A SEX CLUB

ANONYMOUS

I work the door for a swinger and lifestyle club (aka a sex club). So it's not just swingers—it's for anybody who's into any kind of fetish or kink. We welcome all. I work there twice a week, Friday and Saturday nights. I handle security and make sure everyone is safe while they're in the club having fun and getting their rocks off. We serve crudités and fruit platters, but people bring their own liquor to the bar, where the bartender will serve it to you. We don't allow any drug use on the premises. There's different music on each floor, and usually the bartenders choose the music: EDM, rock and roll, like that. Some nights we have a policy that you have to be naked; you can only wear a towel.

There's one room that I warn people about: it isn't for the faint of heart. It's pitch dark and there's gonna be all kinds of hands on you. People usually say they won't go in there, but by the end of the night they've tried it.

I get hit on a lot there. I have to turn down random females all the time. Me and my dick aren't always on the same terms. He doesn't always agree with my decisions.

There are a few websites dedicated solely to swingers, and a lot of people google those and stumble upon our club. That's how I found it. I was trying to find a part-time job, and bouncing is a good way to make money. Somebody suggested I work in a gay club because they tip very well, but I couldn't find a job in a gay club. So I was like, *Let me go even further,* and I googled swinger's clubs. There are quite a few parties in New York, and this place called me back right away. I walked in for an interview and they offered me the job in five minutes.

It's been a pretty interesting job. Every day is a surprise. You probably make an assumption of what and who you might see—and there's a little bit of that—but mostly it's people you would never expect to show up at a swinger's club. There's lawyers and doctors and professors and schoolteachers. People range from the smallest of the small to the biggest of the big. All kinds of bodies. All types. All colors. There's a couple—they gotta be about seventy. The lady will come in and have sex with as many dudes as wanna have sex with her, while her husband takes a nap a few feet away.

There's one girl who comes in every night, and I always tell her she should go pro. She comes in at the beginning of the night and leaves when we close, and she has sex with as many dudes as will have sex with her. She works for the government.

The craziest thing that happened to me there? There was a big dude I patted down—taller than me, bigger than me—who walked in with one of those double-headed dildos, about two feet long. So I make a comment like, "Aw, my man, you came prepared." So he comes in and walks around and just keeps walking. The guy walks by me ten to twenty times in the first hour he's there. One of my coworkers points out, "I think you got a fan." And the way the first floor is set up—if you're standing in the doorway of one of the rooms, you can look directly at me. So this guy was fucking himself in the ass with the dildo, jerking off while watching me. Peeking his head out the door so he could see me. The first time it happened, it threw me. But this guy comes back every other week or so, and does the same thing every time. He will just stand in one of the rooms watching me and fucking himself in the ass. And now I'm used to it. He never speaks to me—even when I'm patting him down. He never encroaches on my space. He just goes in the room and stands in the doorway and has at it.

There's another guy who likes people to walk on him aggressively. Men, women—he likes it all. Every time he comes, people are stomping all over him. He doesn't speak to anyone, he doesn't say a word. He comes in, gets naked, lies on the floor, and gets stepped on until he's had enough. *Stepping on* is a thing. Another guy will sit on the floor and let ladies and guys kick him and step all over his balls, the harder the better. He will orgasm multiple times from it, especially if the lady is wearing heels. He begs them to grind their heels into his crotch.

I've always been the kind of person who's like, *If it's not hurting someone, I don't care what you do.* I'm not judgmental. And it helps for this job. At this club I've learned about so many kinds of things I had no idea existed. I've gotten to the point where I'm like, *Oh, okay.* That's the biggest reaction you can get out of me. If that's what floats your boat, that's what floats your boat.

There's this one woman, way over six foot tall, over 250 pounds. Every time she comes in, she comes in with a full meal—appetizer, entrée, dessert. She comes in with this small guy—five-three, tops. They park themselves in the corner, and they have sex doggy-style while she eats the meal the whole time. I know people incorporate food into sex, but this is a unique way of doing it. The whole time she goes, "Oooh, it's so good, it's sooooo good." And I'm not sure if it's the food or the sex that she's moaning about. If I was him, I'd be like, *She talking about me or the food?* I've seen things that I've never seen before, but that's the only thing that throws me for a loop each time.

Where I grew up is very homophobic. Black people in the hood are very homophobic. I grew up in the hood in the Bronx. Like, if you said something—sometimes not even sexual in any way—people will be like, *No homo!* I've never been on that trip. My mom's cousin is gay, so it wasn't something foreign to me or taboo. Like, how could I talk shit or disparage something that doesn't seem like a bad thing? My mom's hairdresser—he was a very hood dude—but he had long nails and long hair and dressed like a woman. I don't know how he identified. He was part of my life.

I worked at another club before this, and every other Monday they did a swinger's night. Those parties were more fetish-oriented. It was more of a BDSM kind of thing. We have BDSM at our club now, but those parties were solely that. They got crazier than our parties do.

There's been times—as a bouncer at a "regular" club—where I've put hands on people. But not here. The people at this club are very chill. And really, as a bouncer you're supposed to be able to spot things early. Your awareness has to be higher than everyone else's. When I bounce, I say, "Yo—they're not paying me enough to fuck you up!" People laugh, but they get it. And people generally don't want any problems. In a place like this, they're not there to make trouble. When I've had to throw people out, I just say, "Come with me," then I walk them to the stairs and they leave. They don't want to fight.

Sometimes people are just being inappropriate. A lot of the dudes who come are socially awkward. They don't know how to talk to women. So they come to a place like this and they'll see someone else doing something and their first move is to just pull their dick out, hoping to be invited into the action. And that's not really how you do it. So I'll be like, "Yo—back up." And usually they do. But if they don't, I'll be like, "Put your dick away, it's time to leave." But mostly they aren't looking for trouble. Because single guys are not welcome at a lot of parties in New York City on a regular basis. Most places don't want single guys because they are a nuisance. So when they find a spot where they can go, they don't want to act up.

It gets real steamy—literally and figuratively. I'm just glad I don't have to clean the place. There's a cleanup crew—they pick up the rubbers and do the laundry. They get paid pretty well, but that's a job I wouldn't want. I just couldn't do it.

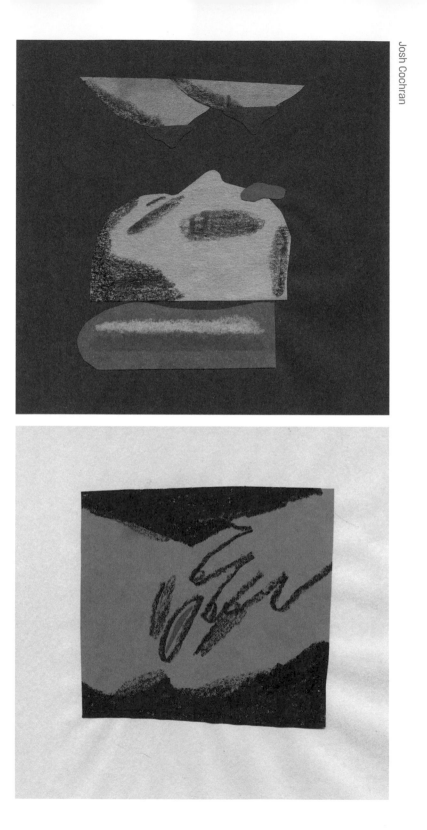

NON-MONOGAMY/ POLY

JULIA Talking to people about this was fascinating. I learned a lot of terminology.

SHAINA Me too. *Primary. Secondary.* Seems like communication is key.

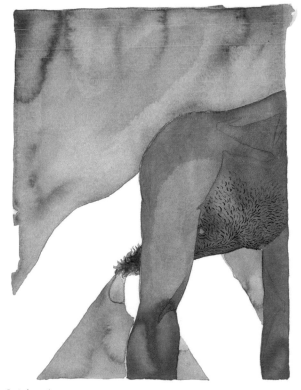

October Joe

I identify myself as ethically non-monogamous. **It was always a battle for me to be monogamous.** I would date multiple women and then think, *This is the wrong thing. Don't do that.* And then I learned that as long as I tell them up front, it's okay. I've always liked a lot of attention from a lot of women because it makes me feel good about myself. So now, telling people ahead of time, I'm able to do it less vindictively.

Except sometimes I explain everything to them up front and they're absolutely fine with it, and then suddenly they're not. For example, I've gone on some dates with people, and I explain my situation and how I feel, and they say at first, "Yeah—totally okay." Then they forge a relationship, fall in love, and suddenly it's not okay anymore, and then I become the dick. It's not a humble brag. I'm now having to say, *You're not being honest with me at the onset. You should make sure you really are okay with it and not just tell me that so I'll date you.*

I identify as poly. Right now I'm seeing two men and also have random hookups. I'm also part of a poly community. It's the lifestyle I want to practice. I don't think love is a finite thing. I believe that you can experience love from multiple people at once. And also it's sort of unfair and unrealistic for one person to fulfill all your needs, emotional and physical.

The cons of being poly are that it takes a lot of time explaining this to people who aren't poly. They think it's just about the sex and that I want to fuck everyone. That's definitely not the case. I also have to take my sexual health into more consideration, especially if my partners are sleeping with other partners regularly. You want to make sure there are boundaries established. You have to get really, really good at communication (which is actually a pro, not a con), but it's very uncomfortable. I've not mastered it. I'm still learning.

If you're going to try it out, my advice is go out there with an open mind and no expectations. Read books about it. There are so many forms of ethical non-monogamy. Have fun with it. Approach everything as play and with curiosity.

Jealousy is not innate to me. I know a lot of people who go through jealousy. You need to recognize that's a you thing, not another person thing. And it's about figuring out where it's coming from—insecurity in your relationship, or the other person is getting attention you would like to get—and communicating that.

Virginia Zamora

I was dating my ex-girlfriend and we were with another couple. And the girl from the other couple was like, what if we were poly? I didn't really know what that meant. In my twentysomething head I was like, *Y'all wanna get naked and fool around? That sounds awesome!* But then it became a relationship, and my girlfriend had become what's called my *primary* and the other girl was my *secondary*. These are poly terms. And then the other guy was just, like, my homie.

Sometimes we'd watch our girlfriends hook up, sometimes we'd get involved. There was a lot of discussion, like, "Is this okay? I'm gonna grab it. I'm gonna stick my face in there, is that okay? Can I lick you down there?" There was a lot of talking. And sometimes there were oversteps and you had to have a conversation.

I'm not a jealous person, so it was easy for me to do. I was secure in my relationship at the time, and I liked the challenge. It was this cool, difficult thing we could do with a great reward.

Group sex is pretty wild—and it's complicated. It was very consent-driven, but sometimes it was really organic. There was this one time when we were in a house in Long Island and the four of us were playing pool. And my secondary asked to give me a blow job and I was like, *Well, this is amazing—sure!* And so my secondary gets on her knees, and she puts my whole member in her mouth, and the other guy was across the room watching. And then my primary started crying and ran away. So I had to take my penis out of the secondary's mouth, and then we all spent a couple of hours talking about it. And then we just went right back to it, and it was fine! I think I was able to make my primary feel good because I said to her, "Look, this is like the bonus level in Mario: you don't need it, but it's fun. I'm just so happy that we get to do this together!"

I like having difficult conversations. I get a certain energy from it, and my heart rate goes up. It turns me on.

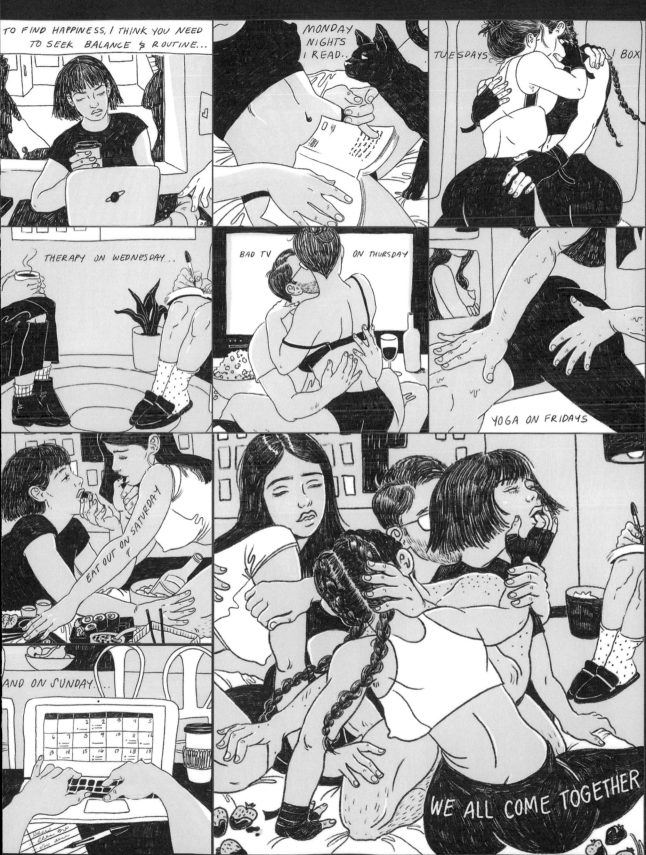

GROUP SEX & SEX PARTIES

JULIA Have you ever been to a sex party?

SHAINA I don't think so. I'd probably remember if I had. I've had some threesomes, though. But they've been very tame.

JULIA What's a *tame threesome*?!

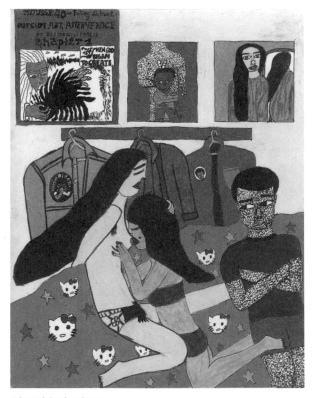

Edward Cushenberry

We met this couple on a beach in the UK. It was all planned. We'd planned it on a website. We turned up on this nudist beach. Me with my partner and these two other couples. There was a windbreak on the beach, so we were all secluded in there, and we all got naked. We all went around and said what we wanted to see and do. The women all started having sex with each other, and this one woman—not my girlfriend—she could squirt and she starts squirting. So we were on the sand performing oral sex with each other. It was unbelievable. We finished it off with me and my girlfriend having sex right there on the sand while the other two couples watched. **My knees kept sinking into the sand. It's very hard to have sex on a beach.** But it was unbelievable. It was a lot of fun.

My girlfriend and I got invited
to a sex party. It was this house
upstate. We got there and
everyone there was gorgeous.
And I was there with my hairy,
dumpy body. I got very anxious.
My girlfriend and I were like,
What do we do? We didn't really
know the etiquette. So at one
point my girlfriend and I hooked
up on the bed in front of everyone,
which was cool and kinda exhibition-y.
But for the most part, we didn't
do anything. We stayed the night,
and the next morning we just
raced out of there.

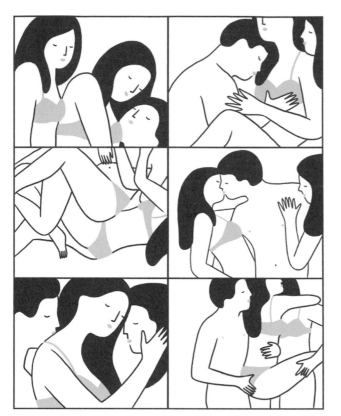

Agathe Sorlet

So it was me and my ex-fiancée. I wanted to spice things up. I knew my girl's friend was bisexual, and I knew she was into my ex-fiancée, so I told her that. So I arranged a night and we all went out. **And I told my ex-fiancée—break the mold, touch her, talk to her, do things I do to you.** So she did. It was one of the best things that ever happened. It was a good threesome. And eventually they kicked me out; they kicked me out of my own threesome! We went on to have nine more of those.

I had a threesome. It was weird. I did it for my boyfriend. He met her. He introduced me to her. It was the first time I had done it. I thought, *I really love this guy, let me just try this out.* I was trying to get into it, pleasing one partner but then not knowing how to please the other. She starts coming toward me, and I'm like, *Ahhh, wait a minute! Work on him first—just let me watch.*

She was cute, but I just don't feel like that toward women. **I watch porn, but it's different when it's real life.**

I stopped into a sex dungeon. I didn't know it was gonna be an orgy. I went to the back room and it was dark. Someone was masturbating, so I started to as well. Next thing I know, there were twenty or so dudes standing around in the dark jerking each other off.

Someone passed me something in a box to sniff. I did, and it was fine. **I didn't know the etiquette of a circle jerk, so I just kind of exclaimed, "I'm gonna blow!"** People moved away and I ejaculated. I think I must have been the first.

I bowed out and shuffled off to the bathroom, holding my pants up and my shirt away from my penis. The lights were very bright in the bathroom. I cleaned up and made my way upstairs to go hang with friends and not speak of this occasion until now, eleven years later.

Farshid Shafiey

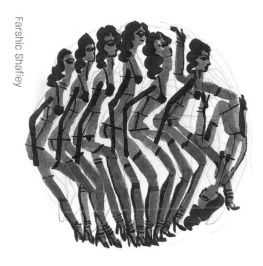

I was born and raised Jehovah's Witness. I have a twin sister. **After puberty, we took totally separate routes.** She met a guy in church at sixteen and married him and has a child. The other day we were FaceTiming and she goes, "Imagine having sex with the same person forever. You've had sex with more than one person, right? I wish I had experienced more people."

Then she asked, "What's the craziest thing you've ever done?"

Well, I dated a guy in college for two years, and a year in he asked, "Would you have a threesome for our one-year anniversary?" I broke down and cried. I said, "No way."

Fast forward another year, and I'm getting ready to break up with him. I was in Sweden, his hometown. One of his friends was super-cute—a girl. I decided *All right, let's have this threesome, and if I don't feel anything afterward I'll know he's not the one.* It lasted five hours. It was amazing. The day after, I called my mom. I told her, "Mom, I had a threesome. And I don't love my boyfriend anymore." I broke up with him, but I still stay in contact with the girl I had a threesome with. That was three years ago now. I had one other threesome after that.

I've been pretty open with my current boy-friend about that. I would like to do it and not have it break us apart. I find the female and male body just as attractive. It just so happens that I fell in love with a guy. I love threesomes now, I guess.

I had a threesome with two dudes once. It was really spur-of-the-moment. I was in South Carolina and out with a coworker of mine. We got a little twisted. She was upset about something, and I was trying to calm her down. These two dudes came up to us. I was like, "Heyyy," because I wanted to have fun. I just wanted the experience for my bucket list. Scratch that one off.

First we got a bottle of Fireball, you know what I mean, gotta get it started.

We went to a hotel. The most thrilling part was, I was the centerpiece. I was getting all the attention. They were both working on me. **You just sit back and relax and let it go.** I gave one oral while one was doing oral on me. Then we would switch positions. I would do oral while the other was doing doggy-style. Just finding different ways to keep everyone involved. Keep everyone happy. It went on for a few hours. One tapped out by the shower. Then, when I woke up—actually, the housekeeper woke me up—I was there by myself.

I don't remember the guys' names. This was five years ago.

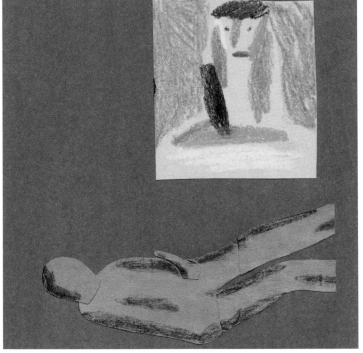

Josh Cochran

I used to live in a small town on the West Coast. It was a really, really small town—not a lot of people. **And there was this social club where they used to have sex parties, and they used to post flyers for it everywhere.** Like where you'd see flyers—as in, *This band is playing!*—there would be flyers for this sex party. Anyone could go. It was kind of unique in that way because they allowed single men, and you could bring your own drugs and booze. Which was really atypical for this kind of thing.

My partner at the time was really into it. She was stoked— she really wanted to go. And it was like this community of people who were really sex positive—some people weren't into having sex at the party, they just wanted to get together and talk about BDSM or polyamory. So I was like, *All right—let's go.*

So we went.

I wasn't expecting to recognize so many people there: A few of my coworkers were there. My boss was there. One of my old classmates was there. That was kind of unsettling, because people were out there, ready to get their game on—whip each other and get on this weird piece of sex equipment and do their thing. But the weirdest thing was seeing my coworkers really going at it.

At the party, everyone was really friendly and outgoing and like, *Hey, what's up?!* But when you get there you have to sign a waiver saying this is anonymous and we won't talk about this outside. So the next day I go to work and my boss was there, and my other coworker who my boss was fucking was there. And it was really weird because, you know, I'd seen all their fucking parts and everything. And I could tell everyone wanted to talk about it, but nobody would outside the party. But there was definitely a lot of winking going on.

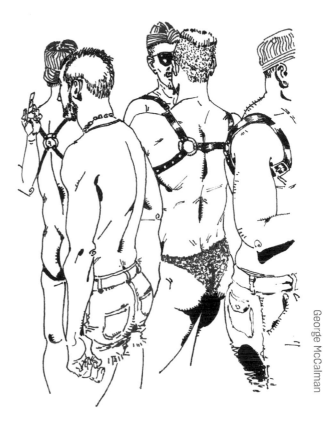

There's a Sunday-afternoon sex party in Paris. It's a piss party. **The advertisement directly translates from French to English as "the most humid afternoon in Paris."**

I fell into this party one day. There's usually some really cute guys who go wearing Speedos. Then there's old disgusting guys literally lying on the floor near the bathroom, waiting to be pissed on. There are no urinals—it's just a trough. This one guy just lies in there. That's the scene of this party.

The last time I was there, I ended up hooking up with this short, geeky guy. Great body. He had really thick glasses. He had great pecs. I love all of these things. Perfect combination. We start going at it. I had actually taken not one but two Cialis before the party. I have erectile dysfunction, and I have a problem getting hard if I'm drunk. So anyway, we're having sex, what you would call *flip fucking*—taking turns fucking each other.

I'm unable to have a pleasurable sexual encounter without poppers, so I do poppers—a hit up my nose. It's like huffing. There's a quick rush, then it relaxes your sphincter muscles. (Quick note: you're never supposed to mix poppers and Viagra or Cialis, because they both lower your blood pressure, but I do it anyway.) So I'm fucking this guy and suddenly everything goes black. I lose my breath and I am instantly soaked in sweat. I remember I pulled out of the guy and was holding onto the stairs for dear life. I can't breathe, and I feel like I'm dying. I crawl up to the main level and order a Perrier. I get another. I sit there for twenty minutes. The guy comes up and finds me. He clearly has no idea anything is wrong, and starts kissing and petting me. I finally compose myself, and then we go at it again.

Lesson learned, though: don't mix those drugs.

A TASTE OF THE MEAT RACK!

BY TURDLUV

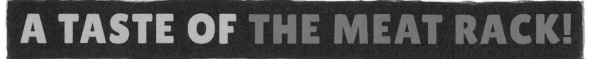

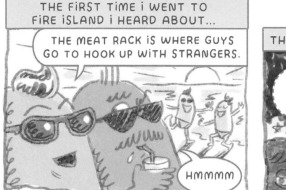

THE FIRST TIME I WENT TO FIRE ISLAND I HEARD ABOUT...

THE MEAT RACK IS WHERE GUYS GO TO HOOK UP WITH STRANGERS.

HMMMM

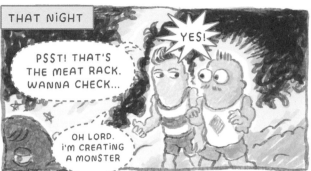

THAT NIGHT

PSST! THAT'S THE MEAT RACK. WANNA CHECK...

YES!

OH LORD. I'M CREATING A MONSTER

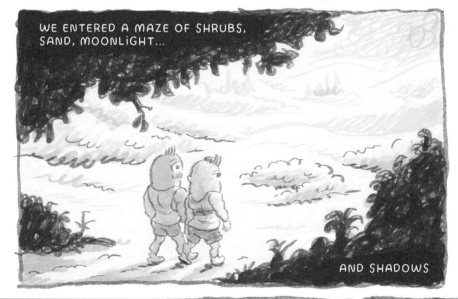

WE ENTERED A MAZE OF SHRUBS, SAND, MOONLIGHT...

AND SHADOWS

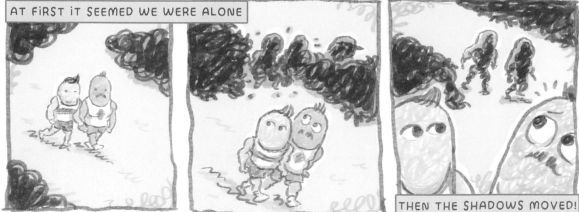

AT FIRST IT SEEMED WE WERE ALONE

THEN THE SHADOWS MOVED!

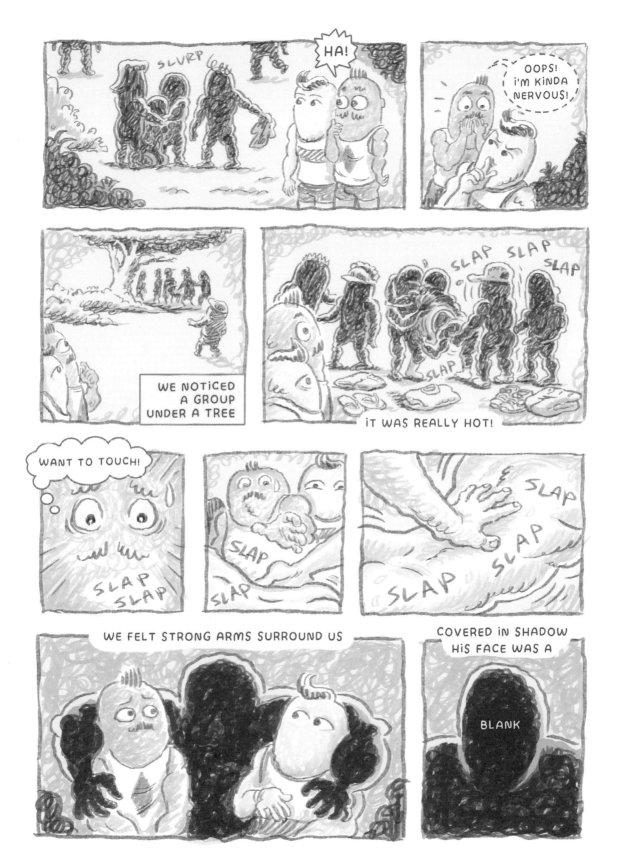

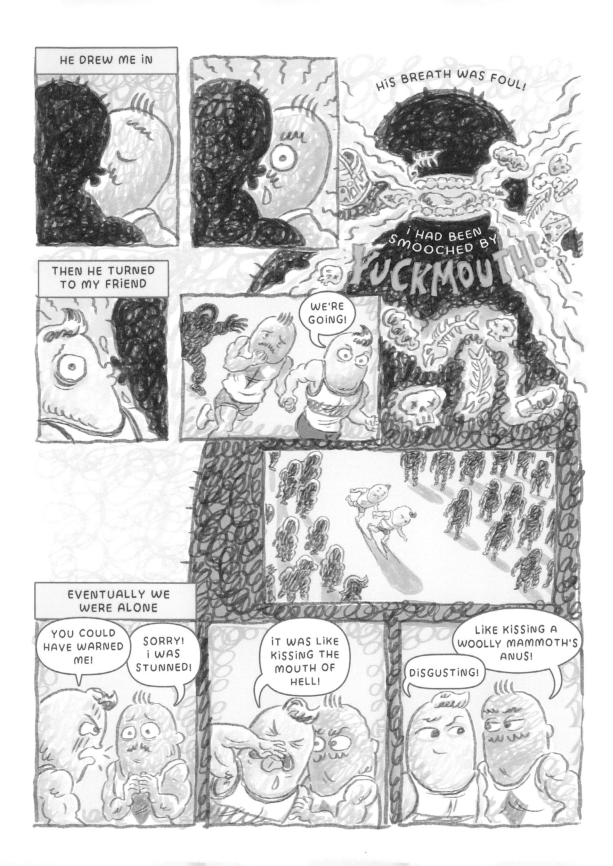

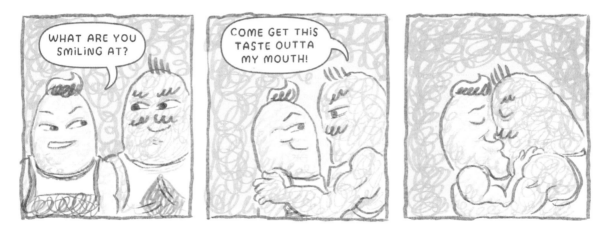

WE LOOKED AROUND US...

WE HEARD THE GENTLE RHYTHM OF THE OCEAN.

WHAT ARE YOU SMILING AT?

COME GET THIS TASTE OUTTA MY MOUTH!

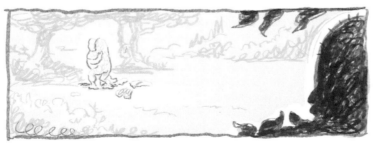

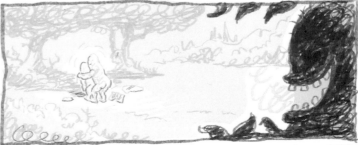

END

Bringing Up Daddy

by **JUDE DRY**

As long as I have been queer, I have been a daddy. But I didn't always have the word for it. Language is sticky for queer people. We're self-aware before we know how to vocalize our desires. When I first came out, I struggled to connect with the words *lesbian* and *gay*; they felt clunky and foreign. Now I like all the words. I'm a genderqueer-butch-dyke-daddy-boy-trans-masculine-of-center-guaranteed-good-time.

But you can call me daddy.

I figured out I was a daddy when I lucked out with my first sex party: a wild queer fantasia where I watched a friend squirt into a pool of glitter and witnessed something called an "octo-pussy"—though it involved only five pussies. In an effort to impress my date, Genn, I let her tie me to a cross and flog me so hard I couldn't sit down for days. I tried two new things that night: subbing and Christ.

I met Genn, or Mistress Maude, on a fetish website where I had specified in my profile that I was looking for a submissive to call me daddy. "It seems like our interests might align," her message read. "Care to meet up and see if we have chemistry?"

Genn was a goth dominatrix who told me she had chosen her name—I suspected her real name was Jen—which was fine by me. She was a punk-rock smoke show in cheap leather and red lipstick—I would've fucked her even if her name was Kevin. She wore all black and took me to goth night at the Pyramid Club, a New York institution and a last holdout of the real East Village. I was so into her that I started wearing leather bracelets. They were subtle.

On our first date, Genn asked how big my cock was. I blushed, trying not to let on that although I'd bought my strap-on years earlier, I hadn't actually used it *with* anyone yet. I definitely didn't want her to catch on that, while I had fantasized about it ever since I first started humping my teddy bear in the loft bed of my childhood bedroom, no one had actually called me *daddy* before.

As Mistress Maude, Genn worked at a midtown dungeon, crushing balls in black stilettos and pissing on suits during their lunch hours. Despite the events of the kink party, in private she was a true submissive. And she loved daddies.

I tried to hide my nerves when Genn showed up at my apartment for our first playdate. Not only was she one of the hotter girls I had dated, I didn't know how to transition from awkward small talk to the daddy portion of the night. How do you order someone to spread their ass when you've just politely offered them a glass of wine? As I was running through potential lines in my head, Genn mercifully interrupted: "I think you need to spank me, Daddy. I've been a bad girl."

My stomach jumped, my chest filled with false bravado, and a current shot down my arms into my hands, now shaking and sweaty. As a devilish grin spread across my face, in my most sultry and assertive voice I said:

"Take off your panties. Slowly. Good girl. Now bend over and show Daddy your ass."

She did. She did everything I said. It was incredible. For the first time in my life, I felt completely free to do or say any filthy thing that popped into my mind.

"You're a dirty little whore, aren't you?"

"Yes, Daddy."

I spanked her ass until my hands stung, leaving splotchy red marks on her pale cheeks.

"Please fuck me, Daddy. I need your fat cock inside me."

I slapped her pretty face, her deep-red lipstick smeared across her chin. "You'll get this cock when Daddy's ready to give it to you." I had met another pervert—maybe even pervier than I.

Genn moved to Toronto to live with her previous long-term daddy, an older butch with gray hair and a not-so-butch name: Emma. I felt envious of my rival—though Genn's mid-thrust comment that I had "a lot of stamina" made me pretty sure I could take her—but I also saw in Emma my rosy future. She was clearly killing it.

After Genn left, I was heartbroken. I took pensive walks, toggling between my sex playlist and my love playlist—Beyoncé singing "Punish me, Daddy," Billie crooning "Good Morning Heartache." I felt like a kid again, infatuated with this elusive woman who had cracked something wide open inside me. Genn empowered me to revel in my sexuality in a way I never knew I could—to dig down into the sludge, without judgment, and pull out something radiant. Something that was once calcified was breaking into glitter.

By their nature, taboos are sexy. In *daddy* we find many of the most provocative fetishes folded into a single word: age play, incest, consensual non-consent, power play, dominance, submission. As a feminist, I would be lying if I said I never feel conflicted about having such base fantasies. But I also know the difference between fantasy and reality. It's one thing to fantasize about letting the overly friendly dudes at the bar gangbang your girlfriend, but no one actually wants it to happen—except maybe the dudes.

Genn may never know the impact she had on me. But I like to think I spread whatever she unleashed in me far and wide. Since then, I've had relationships that explored the *daddy* dynamic deeply, and I've learned how much nasty I need and what is too much. Some days I'm content with an offhand *daddy,* like the way Etta James slips it into the end of a particularly sultry phrase. Other days I long for another Genn, a pervy sub who pushes me to go even darker than I knew I could.

The growing acceptance of the *daddy* meme has made it easier to be out about my fetish, but there's still that little voice inside my head calling me a freak. It's one thing to tweet "fuck me up daddy" ironically, and quite another to call someone *daddy* while they're inside you. I sometimes worry I've given myself this massive handicap: maybe if I liked less oddly specific things, I'd meet people more easily.

But vanilla sex just doesn't do it for me, and I'd rather get off than not. I spent too many years judging my kink, afraid to name it out loud. My friend, the writer and sex educator Betty Dodson, says everyone consents in their fantasies. It's *your* fantasy, so it's all you. Just like dreams.

Daddy holds a special space in the colorful spectrum of dyke/queer/trans culture, with a different meaning for each person. For me, *daddy* is a shortcut to feeling seen in my masculinity. When a femme calls me *daddy,* she's saying, "I acknowledge your sex appeal, even though the world does not." *Daddy* is the big strong man; he's the handsome playboy; he's the cowboy; he's the crooner; he's the prince; he's the hero. He's every part I dreamed of playing as a kid but never got because I "wasn't a boy." He's the guy Etta James is singing about. He's a fantasy. *Daddy* is the drag I never take off. He's my manliness, my tenderness, my sensuality.

Call me *daddy* and you can get away with just about anything.

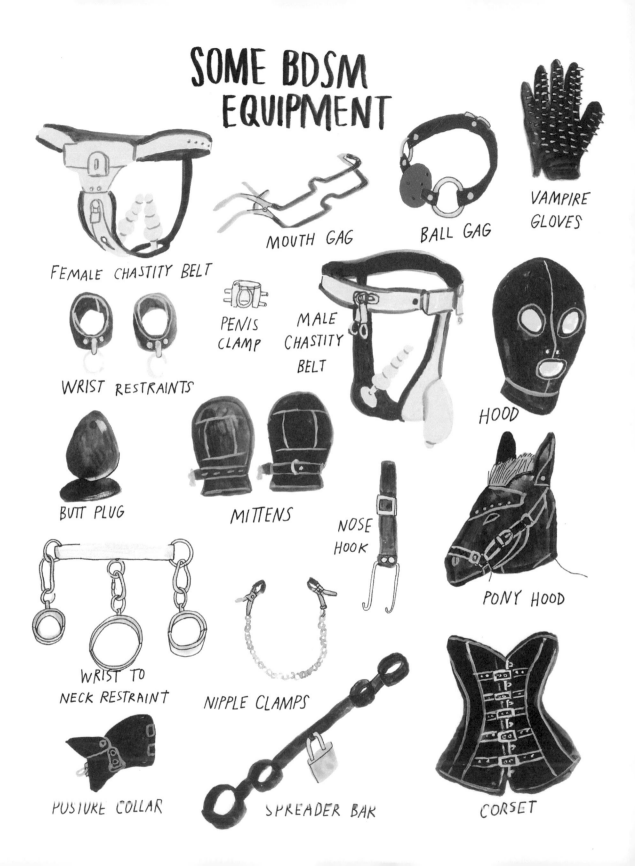

FETISH

JULIA So many heterosexual men told us that they had a secret fantasy of getting pegged by a woman. Meaning that a woman would put on a strap-on and have anal sex with them.

SHAINA Yeah. And every time someone told us, they would say they were so embarrassed to be sharing this private desire with us.

JULIA Like we'd never heard it before.

SHAINA And we'd assure them, you are not alone. We've heard this before. Many times.

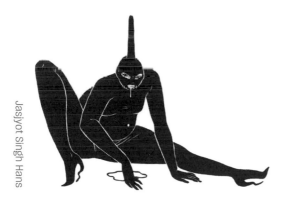

Jasjyot Singh Hans

I love costumes and play. **I have schoolgirl and nurse costumes.** I dated a lawyer once who had me wear a collar and walked me around the house on a leash. I was on my hands and knees. Once in a while he would give me a treat. Then he'd tell me to suck his cock. It was super-fun. I would try not to laugh, but it was a little bit funny.

A girlfriend of mine once peed on me in the shower. She had the water more angled on her, and I was sitting in the bathtub watching her shower. She then stood over my chest and peed on me. **I felt weird about it initially, but then I got mildly turned on.** Then I felt just disrespected—I went through a very quick emotional arc.

It didn't end well, though. I finished my shower alone.

When I was young, I was introduced to choking. I really liked that. You don't know until you try something. And then you learn it's a two-way street, and they can choke you too. Sometimes you're just experimenting in bed and you're like, *Oh, does this feel good?* And something happens and you think, *Oh, I never thought I would like that.* I think everyone should ask, "Can I choke you?" and see if they like it.

I've always been interested in BDSM—with blindfolds and ropes and tying people up next to my bed—but when I met my partner a whole other world opened up. It went from that to whips, floggers, knives, collars, and chains being casual conversation. Like a kid in a candy store, I loved every bit of it and found myself in a master/slave relationship with my partner. The sense of powerlessness I get from being a slave and handing over complete trust turns me on so much.

Let me set two things straight before I continue. **We have a safe word, so I can always stop whatever we're doing.** Second, BDSM and sex aren't the same thing; you can mix them, but that requires consent.

For my birthday, my master took me to a "queer leather" weekend getaway filled with vagina owners and all the BDSM activities you could imagine. They had tops who were open to showing you needle play, fire cupping, whipping, latex beds, rope suspension—practically everything you could imagine. The cherry on top was that sex was allowed, all parties willing. When my master asked me what fantasies I wanted to fulfill, I quietly told them, "A birthday gangbang, sir." I'm usually really shy and have never even had a threesome, but I've always been curious—and I'm not one to half-ass anything.

When we got there the second night, Sir and another person we met (whom I'll call Panther) ran around finding people to be a part of my gangbang. Sir warmed me up, spanking and punching my ass, whispering the dirtiest things in my ear, telling me what a nasty little slut I was for not even caring who fucked me. They lined up dildos and all the toys we had for people to use on me (riding crops, pork-pulling claws, Brillo scrubbers, paddles). Slowly a crowd gathered around me—some voyeurs and some just waiting to be a part of it. I was giggling in anticipation when Panther kicked things off, telling me what a "good boy" I was while I felt everyone's hands on me.

Slowly I felt the scrape of nails, pinching, punching, and light spanks all over my body. All

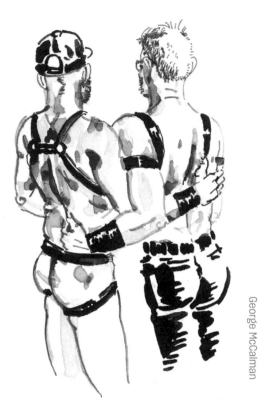

George McCalman

the attention got me dripping and begging to be fucked. After sucking their dildo cock, Panther picked me up by my hips and started fucking me. I felt the people around me getting more aggressive with their punches and hits while Sir watched over everything and egged them on. I couldn't stop moaning, while I could hear people walking up to Sir and asking if they could fist me—which I had never done, but tonight was the night.

People lined up to stick their fingers in me, while Panther said, "Say *Thank you* to [insert name] for fucking you." Every time I screamed their name— "Thank you, [insert name], for fucking me so hard!"—I felt tears running down my face, because feeling someone trying to fit their fist in me felt so fucking good.

The rest of the night left me bloodied, bruised, sore, and used up—but loving every minute of it. They all even stayed after to see how I was, and touched me softly for aftercare. We finished the next night off with an orgy. It was the best birthday weekend I could ask for.

A big thing that's kind of underground in New York's gay community is that a shocking number of gay men have DIY glory holes in their apartments. There are several in a two-block radius of where we are right now. Some of the more elaborate ones have a sheet of plywood with a hole in it, bolted to the entry to their kitchen. **You go into the apartment and stick your dick in this hole, and they are on the other side blowing you.** Others are just a sheet with a hole.

A few around here are very popular. You find the locations on people's Scruff or Grindr profiles. One gentleman I know is so popular that he books people in twenty-minute intervals. His doorman knows what's going on. I'll message him, and he'll be like, *I have someone coming in now; come at 5:20.* I can literally see the person coming out of the building who was there for that, and then I know I can go up. He told me he can service five to seven guys in a single night.

There's something wonderful about completely anonymous sex. You never see their face or know who they are. I'm thirty-three. I'm boring: I go to work, I come home. It's the one thrilling thing that I do. There's this one guy I would go to, and I didn't know he was filming me from his side. You could only see my dick. I accidentally found his videos one day while I was looking at porn. And I found my video because I could hear myself verbally.

I messaged him and was like, "Is that a video of *me*?"

He said, "Yeah—I hope that's okay."

I was really upset for a second. But then I saw how many views it had—and hundreds of positive comments. And I was like, "Oh, I'm okay with that. You can keep it up."

In my early twenties I bumbled my way into a relationship with a girl who was out of my league in both looks and sophistication. **I was always baffled and insecure about why she was going out with me.**

In addition, I was clueless about sex and would orgasm within a few minutes, then immediately fall asleep. Or I would get really emotional and want to sit around sharing an apple and talking about our feelings.

Once, after sex, she told me that her ex-boyfriend used to bring a knife into bed with them and show it to her or sometimes even hold it near her throat while they were fucking.

I gasped and said, "That's awful—I'm so sorry that happened to you!" I thought she was revealing the horrors of an abusive relationship.

She said, "Actually, the knife was kind of beautiful—it was exciting."

I remember I looked at the ceiling and thought, *I don't understand what we're talking about right now.*

Looking back, I think she was telling me she wanted our sex to be exciting, imaginative, dramatic. But even if someone had come in and explained that to me right then in those words, I would have looked at them and said, "I don't understand what you're talking about. What's more exciting than having an orgasm?"

When I was seventeen, I almost lost my virginity to a girl I hardly knew. We had been chatting online via Skype for a few days, where we had met through mutual friends. We hit it off from the start, and not long afterward I—a horny seventeen-year-old boy—steered the conversation into sex.

Turns out she was seriously into submission. Which was great, because I'm seriously into domination. She said she wanted to try bondage and hard physical degradation, despite being a virgin. We laid out a plan to meet at a party on Friday and head back to my house to get it on. Friday rolled around and we met up, then headed back to my place. I tied her up as best I could, and started whipping her with a belt and choking her as "foreplay." (Keep in mind that I was a virgin and had no idea how foreplay was actually supposed to go.) After a few good minutes of wailing on her, I finally go to slide it in. But as soon as I poke the tip in, her whole body goes limp! Turns out she had a pretty low pain threshold, and had passed out from the pain of me whipping her plus putting my dick inside her.

Needless to say, I untied her and took her home, and we never spoke again. I didn't lose my virginity for another two years.

When I was in my twenties, I had this thing with brushing dudes' teeth. Like, whoever I was fooling around with or dating, at some point I'd bring them home, sit them down on my toilet (with the lid down) or on the side of the tub, then sit on their lap and brush their teeth. **I loved the feeling of having my hand all the way inside their fleshy mouths.**

The weird thing is that I was also fooling around with/dating women at the time, but I never had the urge to brush *their* teeth. Maybe it was because I wanted to be inside them. Like this was the easiest/least-smelly orifice I could get myself into with any dudes. Or maybe it was about cleaning them up—I'm not really sure.

Eventually that fetish (I guess it was a fetish) went away, and I wound up dating this guy who I eventually married. He was an alcoholic and had played rugby, so his teeth were either fake or missing. I mean, talk about a crazy mouth! But I never brushed his teeth. Not even once.

I will try everything. Except for anal sex. I make this joke about how I'm saving myself for marriage, but it's kinda true. I've heard a lot of poop horror stories! So I want it to be the perfect situation when I do it.

What I've done in the past is try to send sexy pictures where there's no identifiable marks, because I was always afraid of people showing them to others or putting them online. So I would put fake tattoos on. That way if someone was like, *This is you,* I'd be like, *She has a tattoo that I don't have!*

Sometimes I'd send them to people, and sometimes I'd post them online. Once I put one on Reddit because they have a subreddit where girls post pictures for attention. So I did it and it was nice to get all of these people giving me compliments. On Reddit there were rules, so I couldn't show everything. But when I just send them to people, I show more of my private areas. Sometimes people request things. Your basic requests: *Send me a picture of you fingering your butt.* Stuff like that.

This year I spent some time working in Osaka, Japan, and I took the chance to visit a few Japanese BDSM studios. I connected with one young Japanese woman who had been an exchange student in Seattle, so she spoke good English. I enjoyed plenty of diverse activities, including my first golden shower. We even went to an Ed Sheeran concert together!

For my birthday, she promised me a special experience. I met her at a Starbucks in the early evening, and she took me to what she called a "Happening Bar." After we sat drinking for about an hour, the bar started to fill up with people finishing work, including several groups of women in office suits, some single businessmen, and a few mixed groups, but overall a strong female majority. It just seemed like a normal after-work bar. My friend then said it was time for my surprise and led me through a door into the women's restroom. She told me to strip down to my briefs, then proceeded to use a dog collar and red ropes and other restraints to tie me so that I was immobilized with my head resting over the open toilet bowl.

After making sure I was "comfortable" (so thoughtful!), she left me there, my heart pounding,

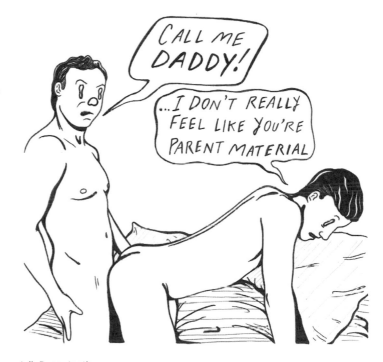

Jaik Puppyteeth

but with a good idea of what was to come. Several minutes later the door pushed open and two office women came in. They squealed in mock horror at finding a foreigner tied semi-naked in the toilet. But then, after a bit of gentle kicking with their shoes, they just lifted their skirts and pulled their panties aside and pissed on me, one after the other, laughing and giggling the whole time while they forced me to drink their pee.

This was repeated every ten to fifteen minutes over the next hour, with women coming in and peeing on my face, in my mouth, and on my body in different ways. Most used their shoes to inflict grazes on my legs

and chest. One drew in Japanese characters on my body with a black marker pen, but all humiliated me by using me as a human toilet. Overall, I drank the urine of at least ten Japanese women while I was there.

My friend came back eventually and untied me, then took me to an adjoining room where I could wash and get dressed again. As we left the bar, I saw a group of women kicking a guy on the ground. My friend explained that it was a bar for dominant women to do what they wanted with masochistic men, and that as a foreigner I was very lucky to have been allowed a glimpse into something that is normally hidden.

Ever since I came across something called pegging I've wanted to try it. I don't know if I would like it, but I'm very curious about it. <u>I like the gender-role flexibility part of it: who is penetrating whom is not set in stone.</u> It's more give-and-take on both sides, instead of just giving and receiving. I want to know how gender relationships are affected in a situation where the woman is penetrating the man, and the man has to open up and receive it. But I've never done it, and I am embarrassed to say I want to.

A *furry* is a person who identifies in some way with an animal identity. There's a huge spectrum of how people identify, though. A lot of furries—but not all—dress up as a way of self-expression. A subset of furries—very few—will wear the costume as a way of showing this is actually who they are. They don't identify even as human.

For me it's more recreational: I believe I have a fox spirit, but I don't believe I'm a fox trapped inside a human's body. I'm a typical red fox; I have tattoos on each arm, a furry name, a white mohawk, and red eyes with blue lining around the irises.

Generally, furries will meet at a "meet" advertised on social media somewhere. Sometimes it's in someone's home. People show up, some people put their costumes on, watch a movie, play games. I organize a meet called a Foxtrot, which we hold at a local LGBTQ bar. We get 250 people. We use *fursuit* as a noun or a verb. People say *getting into suit*.

A lot of people will claim that furry on its own is not sexy. The primary demographic of furry—at least that I see at meets—are gay or queer people. I think the majority are in their twenties and thirties. And that demographic is a sexual one. The sexuality aspect is part of their lives to begin with, and then the fact that they are also furry brings those two together. Sometimes you have sex in the costume, sometimes you don't. The joke among furries is, "Do you have sex in that thing?" One person will say, "It cost $5,000—no way I'm having sex in this!" Another will say, "It cost $5,000—you'd better believe I'm having sex in it!" There's this concept called SPH, for Strategically Placed Hole. A lot of fursuits (including mine) have zippers; you wouldn't notice them. They can be for something as benign as going to the bathroom, or they can be for sex. We pride ourselves on being a freak community—in a good way.

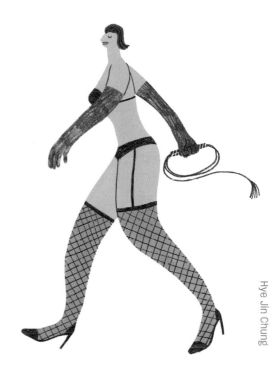

Hye Jin Chung

The main meeting place for furries is the big conventions. There's one in Chicago. There are some in Reno. You can have easily 3,000 furries in the same place. There are hotel parties. Any kind of fetish you can think of, you can extend to furries. You get to put on a costume—not necessarily to conceal your identity, but to have that emotional barrier where you're experiencing it through your character. So there's a level of distance from who you are. You're able to slip into your fantasy and do your own thing as a character that you created; you get to look like the animal you connect to, and do the fetish you're into.

Yes, it's hot in the suit. But if you do it enough, your body acclimates to it. Some people install fans in the head. And there are cooling vests you put in the freezer. I read an article about how this vest made for fursuiting is now being used in the military.

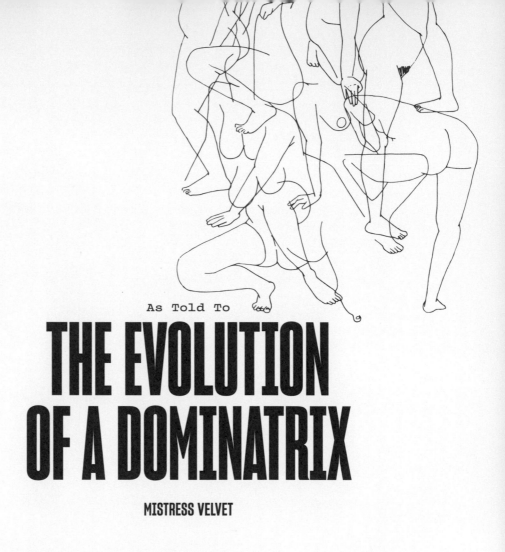

As Told To

THE EVOLUTION OF A DOMINATRIX

MISTRESS VELVET

I am a Ghanaian immigrant, I'm a communist, I'm queer, and I'm a domme. My personal pronouns are *they/them*, but Mistress Velvet—my domme counterpart—is a *she/her*.

Becoming Mistress Velvet was a real evolution for me. When I started, I didn't even have lingerie. I found my first client online. I went looking for someone because I needed the money. I was about to be evicted, and this guy had put out an ask for someone to engage with him in BDSM, and so I got in touch.

I was working as a sex worker. During some of those sessions, I was engaging in some power play. And this lovely person I met doing that really helped me get my business off the ground. He bought me a lot of the items I needed, helped me do the research on how to be a domme, and helped me learn some skills.

One of my biggest memories from back then was doing a session with this sub, and he wanted to be slapped really hard, and I was having a hard time doing it. I would start to go for it, then I'd retreat and scream, "Oh my god! I don't want to hurt you!"

And he said, "You are really nice and so sweet—and because of that you won't make a good dominatrix."

I felt like I'd failed at something. After he said that, I was like *Fuck that, I* definitely *want to do this.* But it was not intuitive for me. I had to learn.

I have my bachelor's in women's studies and my master's in gender studies, with a focus on African-diaspora studies. I was always a straight-A student, and I'm a Scorpio, so I don't like not doing things well. If I'd had no interest in being a domme, I would have let it go. But I *was* interested, so I had to prove to myself that I could do it. I was also very intrigued by the idea of getting to experience a different kind of power. I had never experienced power over men. I had always thought, *I hate the patriarchy,* so it was really good for me to experience this very tangible dominant power.

When folks are reaching out to a dominatrix, they are looking for a specific type of power play within the world of BDSM. Generally, the way we think of a dominatrix is that they are a person who has a lot of power, but really what it is is that we are topping people who want to be submissive. Most of my clients are men, and they feel like they have a lot of power and a lot of responsibility in their regular life, so they come to see me because they want to be submissive and can't find avenues for that.

I live in Chicago now, so I go to a fully stocked dungeon called Chicago Dungeon Rentals. I've also acquired a lot of my own stuff. But I started off in North Carolina, and I didn't have any of that there. There were very few dungeons in North Carolina, so I was domming in hotels. And because of that, I had to get all of my own toys and clothes and paddles.

I pay for a screening service, and there's a reservation form on my website. Each new client has to give me two references from sex workers they've been with before; if they don't have that kind of history, they have to give me information about their jobs so I can investigate them. I have to make sure they aren't blacklisted by anyone. There's lots of boundary negotiations. People tell me what they're interested in, and I have a list of things I will do. There are some things I definitely *don't* do—like cigarette stuff or burning or wrestling or boxing—so I can refer someone to another domme.

Domming is a case-by-case basis. A paddle that I might like for one person might not be right for another. I do a lot of typical obedience stuff: bondage, corporal punishment, spanking, beating, power play, financial domination. Sometimes people want to be blackmailed, so they'll give me their personal information—bank info, Social Security number—and I have to role-play and say, "Give me a hundred dollars or I'll tell your wife you cheated on her!" (whether it's true or not). They just want to feel that loss of control.

I also have a lot of online or long-distance clients, and I'll do things like say, "Send me a picture of you in your underwear or I'm going to dock you $100." I'm finding exciting ways for people to feel punished.

Some people just come and clean my house or run errands for me. One guy acts like he's my chauffeur, driving me around or picking me up from work. That's all that he has the capacity to do because he's married, but it makes him feel useful.

I really enjoy doing puppy play or animal play—for example, sometimes I'll make someone *oink* for me. I try to find humor in how I humiliate my subs. These men are sometimes older than me, and rich, and here I am making them crawl around on the dungeon floor and oink like a pig. It's all hilarious.

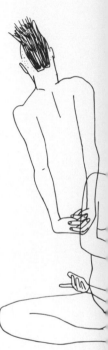

One of my favorite subs would talk about how he didn't even realize how racist he was, and how he had no interactions with black women. He felt a lot of guilt about his privilege as a white man and his ignorance. At first I didn't know how to help him, so I gave him a book by Audre Lorde. I told him to read her because she talks about this kind of thing. Kind of as a joke, I said, "Now write a paper about it"—but then he did! It took both of us by surprise how much he loved doing that. He hadn't read a black feminist text before, and it was exactly what he was looking for.

My domming was budding just as I started grad school, but it wasn't until after I finished grad school that I started having clients read books and write papers. I don't score the papers, but I do offer them feedback.

Now some people request it; others I introduce it to. I have a long-distance sub who I work with, and we are on the phone one or two times a week discussing chapters of this feminist text from the 1970s called *This Bridge Called My Back: Writings by Radical Women of Color*. We go through it chapter by chapter, and we apply it to current society. And he's really applying what he's learning about power, race, class, and gender to his position as a white man.

Recently I had a sub in person, and at the end of our session I gave him an assignment to read a chapter and write a paper for the next time we see each other. So the next time we meet, I will read that paper. I think a lot of people really like the cerebral aspect of this.

I used to do this full-time, meaning it used to be my only job. But now I work at a nonprofit. There's so much work to be done to keep this business going—answering emails, maintaining a social-media presence, and so on. I just recently hired a business manager to help.

I'm married. We have been together for six years. They've been with me through the entire process. One time I had to ask them to come help me out. It's very rare for me to feel in danger, but I had this new client, and he'd had a mistress for most of his life, but she had died five to ten years earlier and this guy was still grieving her. I was the first mistress he had seen since, and he also seemed to have substance-abuse issues. So he showed up at the dungeon smelling strongly of alcohol. Usually this isn't a problem, but he hadn't told me that he would be drinking, and he was very inebriated. He was kind of rude and wasn't going along with things, so I stopped the session and said, "This isn't working—I'm not getting you into the headspace, and I'd like to stop the session." At that point he got really aggressive. No one else was at this dungeon at the time, and I felt very unsafe, so I called my partner and told them the sub wasn't leaving; could they come to help me?

I've been fired from two nonprofit jobs when they found out I'm a professional dominatrix. One of my sub clients who is an attorney said I could make a case, but I didn't want to. It was too traumatizing. But with this current nonprofit job I am doing trainings about sex work, so sometimes I will disclose what I do as a dominatrix. And when I interviewed for the job, I told them right away about my work. I feel no shame about it. I feel a lot of pride about this work.

I think of sex work exactly the same way as I think of other forms of work. There's a lot of misconceptions about sex work. I think some people have a misconception that sex workers aren't empowered at all. I also don't want to romanticize it—because it's not all utopian. But in many respects it's like all other kinds of work—some of it sucks, and some of it is great.

At the nonprofit, I train people to work with sex workers; the goal is to have them listen to the sex worker and determine whether the sex worker likes what they do. If they don't like it, then the goal is to get them out of that work and into other work. And if they are enjoying their sex work, the goal is to see how we can make sure the work is sustainable and safe. There's such a variety of sex work—we always think of sex workers as prostitutes who are murdered on *CSI*. But that isn't accurate. I have a friend who is disabled and in a wheelchair, and she makes porn at home. There are a lot of options for sex workers.

I make substantially more money as a sex worker than I do at my nonprofit job. So for some people, it's a very empowering way to support themselves when they wouldn't otherwise be able to.

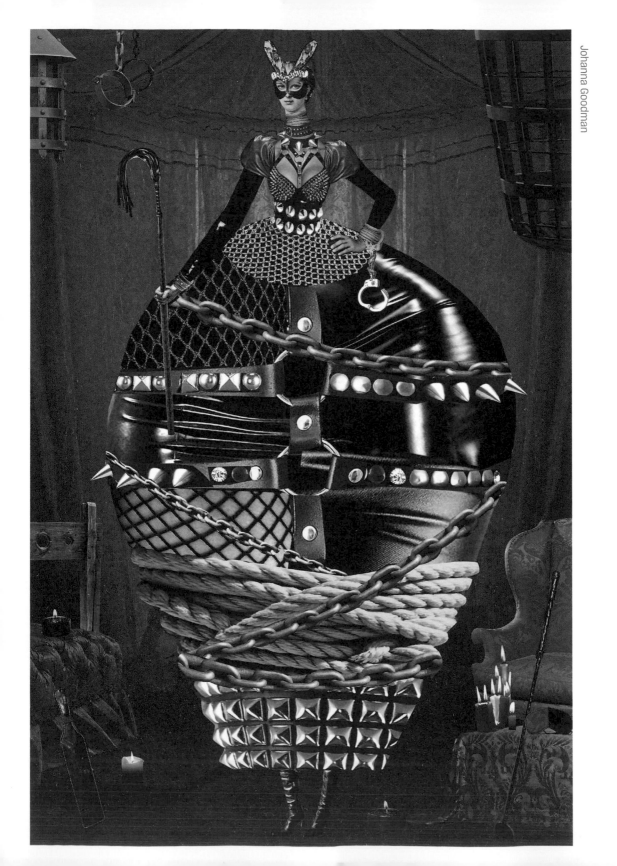

SEX WORK

SHAINA The stories we gathered on this topic ran the gamut from hilarious to intense.

JULIA And it was one of the topics that had the most diversity—we spoke to men, women, gender-nonconforming people, older people, younger people, and so many people of different ethnicities who had done or were still doing sex work.

In the 1990s, when I was in college, I was a male exotic dancer for two years. I was working at a pretty conservative job, wearing a suit every day. I wanted more money. There was an exotic male revue near my apartment in San Francisco, and it kind of intrigued me when I was walking home from work. One evening I ducked my head in and asked what the process was. The manager said, "You come in, you do an audition, and if you do well, we'll hire you." He asked if I wanted to come back next Tuesday, and I told him that sounded good. I went back Tuesday. I danced and was hired on the spot.

I wiggled with rhythm, trying to be sexy. I worked on the pole a little bit. Each dance lasted about thirty minutes. That was your set. My thighs were dead after that. I couldn't do anything afterward. You have a queue of music laid out. I would plan how I wanted my set to be and put in music accordingly. I would be up on the stage for the first song, so that song had really good energy. Then I would go down into the audience for a couple of songs and do up-close work. Then for the last song I would go back onstage and finish off with a bang.

The audience was mostly guys in the early part of the evening. Then, around ten o'clock, girls would come in. I usually worked on a Thursday, Friday, or Saturday night—those were the "gravy"

nights. **You make your money dancing for the guys. It was about twenty to one—literally: you get a $20 tip from a guy and a $1 tip from a girl.** Girls didn't know what they were doing, but guys have been going to strip clubs forever. Still, it was a lot more fun to dance for the girls because I like girls. The bigger the group, the more crazed they were. Guys were not crazy at all. They were much more reserved. I had regular customers.

My stage name was Alex Maxxx. How I got that name was the manager just looked at me and said, "You kind of look like an Alex." And then we added the *Maxxx*. Most of the time, I performed in my suit. I would come from my day job, so that was common for me. I did have a little sailor's outfit I would wear a lot. You take off everything, eventually. (Except for your socks—that's where you keep your dollars.)

When I said finish with a bang, I really meant it. It would end with ejaculating. You have to keep your erection for thirty minutes while you are dancing. It took practice, but you get used to it. I was very fit then. And I have a decent-size cock.

My first week was the week before the dot-com bust, and I made $1,600 a night. After the dot-com bust it would be about $400 for a Thursday to about $800 on a Saturday evening.

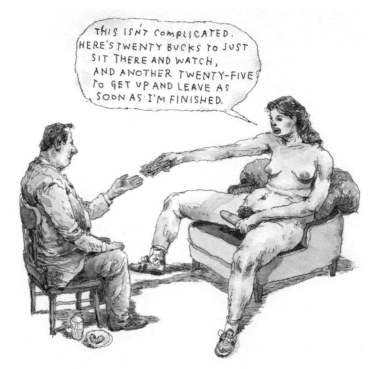

This isn't complicated. Here's twenty bucks to just sit there and watch, and another twenty-five to get up and leave as soon as I'm finished.

I dated an escort for two and a half years. **She challenged my relationship to sex, got me thinking about what constitutes a relationship and sexual fidelity.** She could disassociate sex from love, which I think I do. Ultimately it didn't work out, though.

I supposedly lost my virginity to a prostitute at the age of twenty-six. I had looked her up the old-fashioned way—in the Yellow Pages.

She looked like death as she entered my hotel room. Smelled like it, too. Her joyless face coordinated perfectly with her ugly brown jumpsuit and sickly, pale-white skin. If she told me her name, I don't recall. Didn't matter—not to me, not to her. I assume we exchanged some banal pleasantries before I took off my clothes and lay on the bed faceup. I think she may have removed the top part of her jumpsuit to reveal black lingerie, but that did nothing for me. I was

about as turned on as a branch on a willow tree. She sucked my condom-covered cock with all the passion and excitement of a bored teenager working the register at Walmart.

I closed my eyes and fell back on the only thing that had worked for me up to that point: my imagination. I have no idea what my fantasy was, but it was good enough to make me come. I'm guessing I paid her $75. It was all a poor journalist could afford. After that, I pledged I would never do that again. Little did I know my journey into the seedy sex-trade world was only just beginning.

I had been going to the Russian Baths in the East Village for a couple of years. A *schvitz,* they'd call it. In the honeymoon years of living in NYC, I was drawn to unique spaces and experiences like this. I'd frequent the coed days, because I'd heard of the men-only time and I didn't want that kind of experience. The place attracted old-timers, Orthodox Jewish men, young people with Groupons—all types. The place was hot—the radiant sauna room would singe your nose hairs when you walked into the cavernous and crowded space. I enjoyed leaving exhausted—cleansed and relaxed. I was a different person in a different place.

One couldn't help thinking about sex. The heat would wear you out and stunts the prefrontal cortex. Plus the bodies—glistening, glowing bodies. The sounds of exhaustion from tolerating 110-degree-plus saunas and steam rooms. I loved looking: men's arms, shoulders, backs, legs, ankles, feet. We like what we like.

Two workers—brothers, but they didn't look alike—would do the rounds, asking if bathers wanted treatments. To the frequent bathers, they'd look at you and ask, "Today?" Russian accents, one a swarthy brute, the other thin and wiry. I was drawn to Ilya. Dark hair and eyes, thick muscular build, a long scar on his face.

I'd had a platza treatment before. It's public. They cover your eyes with a cold wet towel, beat you with oak leaves, stretch your joints to their limits, then throw ice-cold water to cool you from the intense heat. You are powerless. It feels good to relinquish control. That day Ilya asked if I wanted a scrub-and-mud treatment.

We went into one of the private metal stalls in the general room. I could hear everyone—the chatter, the laughing, the first-timers figuring out how to use the space. Ilya gave me a scrubdown. It felt rough and exhilarating. He had me turn over from my stomach to my back. He soaped me up. He grazed too close to my dick, and there was movement. What can I do? I'm a gay man. I like men. He noticed it excited me and gave me a puzzled look. It was probably feigned, now that I think of it. I shrugged it off and apologized. He asked if I liked men or women. When I told him the truth he looked confused. "Why?" I told him that that's just the way it is. He laughed and told me that was a good answer. He left me wrapped in warm, wet towels and told me to rest. He'd come back.

I lay there and tried not to be embarrassed. I wasn't, actually. It's funny how sometimes we have shame and other times we have pride in our shamelessness. Nonetheless, I wasn't going to be ruled by hormones and genitals this time.

He came back, unwrapped me, and started rinsing me off. He got closer to it...moving gently and deliberately. Before he even got close to it, I was rock hard. He took it in his hands—soaping it up, retracting my foreskin, massaging the glans, using another hand to rub my thighs. I looked at him and he looked back. He leaned in over me and close to my ear. He asked me if I wanted to come. I was speechless. I barely could nod. He let me play with him. His cock was thick and fat and uncut—one of the many ways I like them.

Needless to say, it didn't take much to orgasm. I had fantasized about this man before, but this was better than any fantasy I had had. When I came—it was an exercise in silence. If I could have, I would have let out a moan from the depths.

Afterward he smiled at me, rinsed me, dried me off, and put me back in robes to join the other bathers. He winked and put an extended index finger to his lips: *shhhh.* I knew what to do. I've kept many secrets.

We used to go to the Clermont Lounge in Atlanta. I'm not sure what it's like now, but at that time it was a very dive-y strip club, and the women who stripped there were very atypical of what you imagine a stripper to be. They were older; they had regular, differently shaped bodies, like anyone you would see walking down the street. Some of them wore wigs. There was one stripper whose specialty was being able to crush beer cans between her breasts without using her arms to assist. <u>She also specialized in slapping guys in the face with her breasts.</u> There was a real respect for these strippers. It felt unique.

I was hustling a little bit, finding money for books and stuff for school. This anonymous man hits me up on Grindr, then calls me and in this very thick accent says he won't send me a face pic, but he will meet me outside my residence.

So I go outside, and to my surprise it's a Hasidic man. **And suddenly my heart kind of melted, because this man was so sweet on the phone and he has this extreme paranoia that I would spread his information or identity and it would get back to his home in Israel.** So I just get in the car. And I say, "Let's go to the Meatpacking District and go to one of those hourly hotels."

So we get there and he wants me to walk far away from him. Then we get to the hotel and he starts getting a lot of anxiety and he says, "We shouldn't do this." And by the way, at that point he's saying he just wants me to give him a massage. He denied he was gay and just wanted a massage.

I told him, "If you're on Grindr looking for a massage, you might have a little gay in you—and that's fine."

So we go in, and I tell the lady that he doesn't have an ID card. He did, but he didn't want to show it. We get in the room and he tells me there are two rules:

Number one: I can't touch his genitals with my hand.

Number two: If he gets "very hot in this area" (his genitals), I should blow with my mouth either on his genitals or in his ass. Literally *blow*.

He got undressed. And I was thinking, *He doesn't feel comfortable with his sexuality, but I do,* and that gave me some power. So while he was getting undressed I asked him if I could wear his kippah

while we're in bed. There I was with this kippah, chewing gum, feeling like *the* prostitute of the twenty-first century. He was gonna pay me 200 bucks for this "massage." I had this weird need to make him understand that he's gay. I kept doing more than he asked for. I kept thrusting my body at him. I turn him around, and as I'm giving him a massage he says he is getting hot, so I'm supposed to "blow."

This super-Hasidic guy, super-Orthodox guy, is on all fours, and I'm blowing on his asshole, and I'm like, "Is this helping?"

And he's like, "Yeah, yeah."

And I'm like, *Let's see what the threshold is for him.*

So I go under him, and I'm blowing on his balls, and I'm like, "Is this helping?"

And he's like, "Yeah, yeah, it's helping."

And then I stick out my tongue and give him a blow job, and I ask him, "Is *this* helping you?"

And he says, "Yeah, yeah—I think this is gonna cool it off right away."

I said, "I don't know if you know what this is, but this is called a blow job, and if a man is giving you a blow job and you enjoy it, you might be gay."

So then he got really mad and got off the bed. He got dressed and said, "You don't think I know what happens in this hotel? You're trying to tell me what I am?"

He gives me my cash and runs out. I get dressed and run after him. And the lady at the desk is like, "Thank god you're alive! That guy gave me no ID, and now fifty minutes later he's running out alone! I thought he had killed you."

I said, "No, I'm alive—I'm alive." And now that guy's probably just back in Israel.

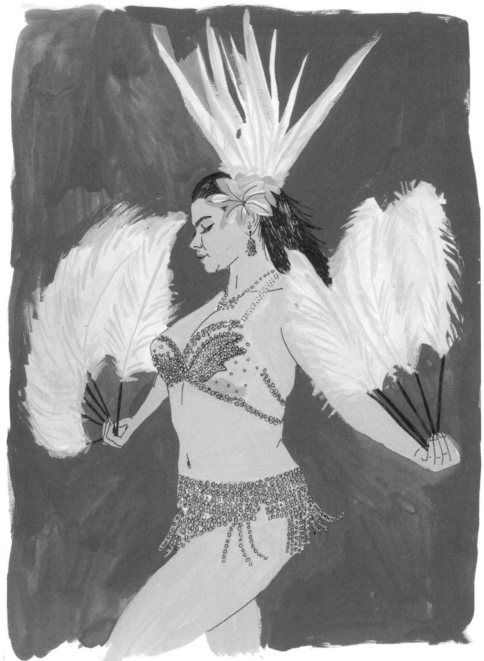

"When I'm onstage, I can be whoever I want and I can express myself. It's freeing and liberating. Burlesque helped me learn to love my body. I realized that when I watch a show I enjoy seeing all shapes, sizes, and colors. I never thought I could be sexy but I learned that confidence is sexy. I carry that with me on and off the stage."
— Tiny D

I've had multiple sugar daddies. It's an exchange of energy. For some people, in exchange for intimacy—connection, talking to someone—they give you money. Most of the time, it's an exchange for sex. I give them sex, and they give me money.

I started doing sex work in 2016, when I graduated from my master's program and realized *Fuck—I have a lot of debt!* I had heard through the grapevine that you could get a sugar daddy. **I had a lot of friends who were sex workers, and I had done some stuff before—I had sold my panties on Craigslist. I was super-desperate for money and couldn't find work, and I have a particular kink for old men.** There's something about them that is taboo and gross, but the masochist in me really likes it. Maybe it's daddy issues, but I've always had this kink. It's how I got off when I was a teenager: I would read the ads on Craigslist that were like, "I'm an old dirty man looking for a barely legal girl." I didn't like porn, but I would read those ads and masturbate.

I had this dawning moment where I was like, *I'm in a good position here: I actually like old men, so I should get a sugar daddy.* So one of my classmates had done a presentation on sugar daddies at school, and I asked her for the website she talked about. You had to have a college email address to be a girl on that website. So I used my NYU email address, and I was like, *Let's do this.* I had zero idea what I was doing, but I set up a profile and started messaging old men and talking dirty to them.

First I would do a phone call to make sure they weren't too creepy. I did a phone call and met up with this guy at Washington Square Park, and we were talking about what he was looking for and what I'm looking for. I was trying to keep it cool and keep my boundaries, even though I knew nothing about this. He was like, "How about $500 every time I see you?" and I was like, "Yes, that's great." (I thought he was gonna give me $100, so I didn't even try to bargain him up.) Anyway, we weren't gonna do anything that day. I just wanted to meet up and suss him out at first. That day he did give

me $100—it was a hundred-dollar bill. I had never seen one before.

I got really scared afterward, and I didn't reach out to him for four or five months. He wanted me to wax or shave my pussy, and that freaked me out because at that point I had never done it before. I had only been with queer people, and they liked my hair. I was like, *No, that's a boundary—I can't compromise on that.*

So for a while I found a different sugar daddy who didn't care about that. This guy lived in a different state. He was pretty young. He was giving me $600 a month. I did everything wrong that you could do as a sex worker: I told him my real name, gave him access to my bank account, gave him all my free time. He basically started stalking me, and eventually that relationship ended.

So I decided to contact the first guy from Washington Square Park. I was like, *Lemme just try getting a wax and contact him.* I did the wax and it was totally fine, and then I met up with him. Before this guy, I had never really done kink. Like my partner and I had been doing kink-lite. But this sugar daddy—he was a freak. He had been doing hard-core BDSM for, like, twenty years. I learned a lot from him. I actually learned that I liked pain. I found out that I liked feeling kinda scared and then getting fucked after that. I loved having sex with this guy. The first time I met with him to have sex was the first time I'd been in a nice hotel. We went to this luxury hotel; it was gorgeous. As soon as we got to the room, he took a pillowcase and made it into a rope, then took my hands, put them behind my back, and tied them. We had made no negotiations yet, and I was scared, but had also made my peace with it.

I was with him for years. I would see him once or twice a week. We had a legitimate kink relationship. He was married, had a kid. He didn't know that I knew who he was, but I figured out things about his life. And then one day he just totally ghosted me. He had been asking me to bring in a younger girl for a while but I didn't, and then eventually he just stopped texting me.

I used to be a burlesque dancer when I was much younger. This is back in the 1970s, in Times Square. **And we'd have live sex onstage.** We'd get undressed onstage little by little, then our male partner would come out and have sex with us onstage. The audience loved it. We'd get $60 per day. You could do it for six or seven days in a row and make some money. We had eight-hour shifts.

I met some big porno people at the time—Annie Sprinkle, Harry Reams. Sometimes we'd travel and go do burlesque at Plato's Retreat, which was a swinger's club back then. It was fun back in the day. They had these booths—the booth would go up and you'd shimmy around while guys watched you and jerked off. It was fun and funny and felt free.

I'm broke. I don't come from money like a lot of the kids from school do. So I went on Seeking Arrangements, looking for a sugar daddy or momma. It's a lot like a dating app. There are profiles. You can say what you want—for example, "I'm a sugar daddy looking for a baby." I have friends who have daddies, and they can do whatever they want and this man pays for it. It was hard for me to find anyone to meet me, though. I think it's because I'm not a typical American beauty. I'm not tall or thin or blond. I think they expect Barbie dolls.

I did connect with a few guys on the app, though—with varying results. Once I met this much older man near Central Park; he was forty-six, more than double my age. I thought he was so handsome. I am usually attracted to older men like him. This guy had all his hair, slicked back. He was in a suit. I was like, *Damn.* But he sees me and he says, "I can't do this. Here's $50. Leave me alone." He paid me to leave and we hadn't even talked for five minutes.

I have a picture on the app, so I'm not sure what happened. He said it was because I looked so young. I still thought maybe I look fatter or uglier in real life. Funny thing is, I actually saw him by mistake two days later. I was walking dogs for money, and I was trying to control one of the dogs, and I look up and it's him. He put on his sunglasses and sped away like he didn't see me. Another time I met a different guy for tea, and he had bird shit on his shoulder and smelled bad, so I left. I didn't even ask him for money. I told him it wouldn't work out.

My third attempt worked out. There was a guy who wanted his balls busted—he wanted to get kicked in the balls. He had never done it before, and I pretended I was experienced. My friend told me I better be careful because I could do real damage. I told my roommate what was going to be happening so she would go away. She thought it was cool. He came over for thirty minutes. **I kicked him in the balls a few times and he gave me $200 cash.** I didn't even have to take off my clothes.

Then he said, "I want to do that every Wednesday."

And I said, "Sure," because it was great money. But I never heard from him again.

Other friends have met their glucose guardians in other ways—like someone reached out to them on Instagram, or found them on Tinder. They get DMs that say, "I just want to pay for you to live." It's incredible.

When I was younger I used to do fetishes for money for a company in Brooklyn. I've seen a lot of crazy shit. The first time, a guy wanted me to show up at his hotel room. **As soon as he opened the door, he wanted me to hit him.** I was like, "I just can't hit you." So I went in, and he had all these crazy things like ball gags. I did well. I liked it and kept on doing it. It starts at $300 an hour.

I'm a BBW (Big Beautiful Woman) but I'm on the smaller size, which is saying something because I'm a big girl. But I heard some guys say I'm not big enough for them. They like for you to step on them with heels on. There was a really skinny guy who used to come see me. He would give me $400 for half an hour. I would wear stilettos. He'd lie on the ground. He'd be jerking off. It was so weird to be naked and step on him. He would hold his breath, and I would stand on his chest.

I had a Jamaican guy, he would put my feet on his chest. While he's stroking my feet, he would be jerking off. Then he'd like to come on my feet. That was his thing. I'm like okay, for $300. Also you have a driver, who'd take 10 percent. At the end of a good night, I'd walk away with $1,200.

I've had a few bad experiences. Not because of the company, but because of the person. Usually, they check the person out thoroughly before, though. I've done everything—threesomes, two girls, swinger's clubs. There was a good swinger's club on Twenty-Eighth and Fifth, Le Trapeze. I used to go there all the time. They had private rooms.

I don't do it just for the money. I like the work. I probably wouldn't do all that for the money.

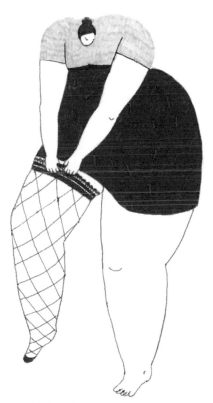

Atieh Sohrabi

SOME SEX SHOPS IN PARIS

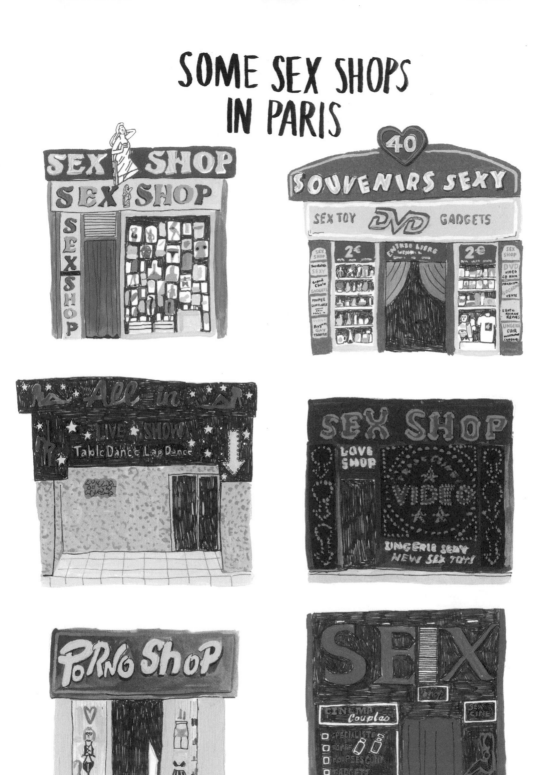

Julia Rothman

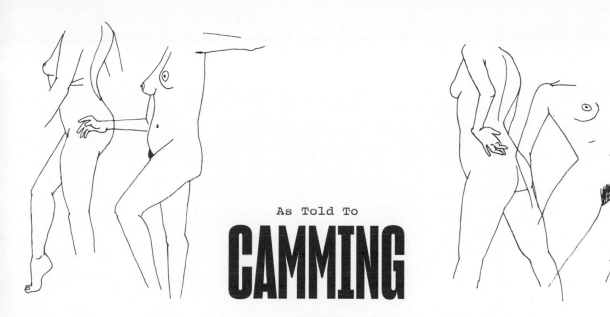

CAMMING

LAUREN DUCK

I'm twenty-two. I live in LA. I've been doing sex work since I was eighteen. Since before I lost an arm. And I continued doing it after I lost my arm. My name's Lauren, but I go by *Duck* online. It's my nickname. I used to have a Twitter account, and the @ was *uglyduck,* then it just caught on, and people started calling me *Duck*.

I'm originally from DC, but my mom and I moved around a lot and I grew up mostly in North Carolina and Maryland. I've never been into academics. I didn't go to college. And I never wanted a nine-to-five job. When I was eighteen, I was trying to move out of my mom's house, and I was like, *What can I do that would make me some money, fast? Something that I would be good at?* I'm very open about my sexuality and my body. Ever since I started having sex, I was just very open and didn't feel any shame, so I thought I would try sex work.

First I tried camming. That's where you're livestreaming your sex work and people can interact with you while you're posting it. It's through a cam site. There's this third party involved, and they take a big percentage, so you're not really working for yourself. That didn't last very long. I stopped camming and just started selling videos to people personally. I was good at it. And it was fast money. I found some success in it.

When I lost my arm, I got even more into it. Actually, I wouldn't have a following if I hadn't lost it.

I lost my arm in 2016. I was nineteen at the time. I was on a moped and I was going too fast—way above the speed limit—and I lost control, slid into the median, and flew off the bike. I hit a street sign, and it sliced my arm clean off. I coped very easily—partly because of my personality, but also having a big support system on social media. All of these people were just so accepting of it, so it made it easier for me to accept it too.

What I do now is not as interactive as camming. I do Premium Snapchat, where people pay to get added and watch the videos I post on there. It's not live. I like it a lot better than camming. It's more independent; I don't have to go through a third party. I get paid directly through Patreon, and I get to set up my own rules and choose who gets to view me. People can message me about my videos, but it's not interactive.

I try to have a relationship with my audience, but it's hard. I have different tiers of viewers. My first tier—the $25 tier—I don't interact with very much. But then it goes up to $100, so I respond to them every single time. The biggest part of why people buy Premium Snapchat, rather than just going to Pornhub, is to have an interaction with someone. Lots of people overseas buy Premium Snapchat. It's mostly straight men, but I also have women who subscribe.

I'll do a series of videos, the longest being five to ten minutes. I do it almost every day. Making up concepts for these videos comes very easy to me: I'll buy something that looks good and put it on, then do things that I'd like to watch. I'll film them and sometimes cut out a couple of things, but usually they aren't edited. Sometimes I play music, sometimes I don't. People really like to listen to me enjoy it. Sometimes I'll talk and tell people what I'm doing, and sometimes I just make noises. I get pretty into it; I'll full-on masturbate. I have dildos that look pretty realistic, and I'll suck on them. I'll make noises because people like to hear that. It's usually just me, but sometimes I'll have another girl make videos with me.

People don't judge me for doing sex work in LA. So many people I know in LA do sex work. Most people I hang out with I'm meeting off of Twitter; they already know this stuff before I meet them, so they're not judging me, which makes it easier. But when I find someone to date on Tinder, I do worry that they will be judgmental or mean. I tell people pretty quickly—usually after seeing them three or four times. At first, though, I tell people I'm a content creator or a social-media influencer; I don't want to jump right into it. If I wasn't familiar with the scene, I don't know how I would react, so I ease in.

It's one of the least big deals in my life. I don't really think about it as taboo or anything. It seems so normal. I have surrounded myself with people who do the same thing, and I've been doing it for so long. Very rarely do I have bad interactions with people over it. Online, some people are dicks about it; people will make fun of me for being a one-armed porn star, but it's nothing that could actually get to me. And my mom's side of the family is extremely supportive about it. They are a super-conservative Southern family, but they've been so kind about it. They unconditionally love me, so they support me no matter what. But my dad and his wife are not.

In real life I have a lot more insecurities, and I am not as comfortable as what I put out there. Still, what I'm doing on Snapchat isn't a character—I just don't feel insecure on Snapchat (unless I've eaten a lot and I'm really bloated). I just feel more confident because I can dictate my angles, I can dictate how people see me. When I'm having sex with people in real life, I can't control how they see me, and that causes some insecurities.

I want to do sex work for as long as I can. I don't ever plan on doing actual porn, but I like doing these videos. What I do doesn't require too much from me. Sometimes what I do feels like I'm stuck in a rut, and I don't leave my house because I can do everything from home. I'd like to have a job where I get out of the house and talk to people. I'm about to move to Portland, and I plan on getting another job, just to have something to do and have something to fall back on in case this ends sooner than expected. But I don't think it will.

I stopped doing sex work for two months because I had some medical issues, so instead of my normal content I was posting pictures of my dog. Once I felt better, I started posting about my sex work, and all of these people were like "*What?!* I thought this was a dog account!" I lost two thousand followers. But eventually I got other followers who were into the sex-work stuff.

One of the things that I don't like about sex work is devotees—people who solely want to see my content because I am missing an arm. That is something I still don't know how to deal with or how to talk about. I don't have much respect for their kink; it's a little weird to me. They will ask for videos of me putting on a prosthetic arm and taking it off—shit like that. I don't do it. I find it kind of gross. It's a niche group, but there are enough people in it to make it weird sometimes. I say to them, "If you wanna see that, you're gonna have to pay me a lot more money."

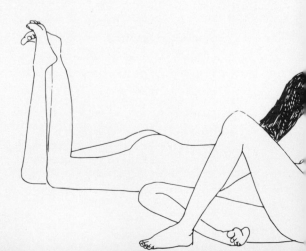

SEX TOYS

SHAINA In college I worked as a cleaning woman, and I saw so many vibrators. It was eye-opening. Mine was this boring purple one, but people had all kinds. It was inspiring.

JULIA What was the most common kind you saw?

SHAINA A penis on one end and a thumb on the other. I saw a lot of those.

My then-boyfriend once got me a big bag full of sex toys for Christmas. I was not impressed. Massive glass dildos and lube. Not only that, but he worked in a sex shop, so he got it all as a rush lot on Christmas Eve. He is now my husband, and needless to say he is still sorry. **Do *not* give your partner massive dongs in year one of a relationship.**

When I went to college, my aunt was like, *Don't have sex.* She was like, *Get a vibrator and masturbate.* So I ordered one online, and it showed up at my dorm. I was immediately like, *This is lit!* I loved it. It was a bunny rabbit, and it would go inside you and swirl around. **I'm a girl who always has a vibrator; I have two right now.** I've broken them before, too. I have a strong vagina.

I started working at a sex store in March, and in April my boyfriend of two years dumped me. Working in a sex store is less fun when your heart and sex drive feel trampled and deflated.

On a standard shift, I help single people find vibrators for solo play, but mostly I help couples or coupled people find toys to enhance their mutual pleasure in bed. **While I am still genuinely excited to help them and listen to their needs, I am struggling to summon the camaraderie I felt before.** Now, in the slow hours, I wander around the store thinking about the ways I would have liked to use the partner-relevant toys and trying to decide if I need a new vibrator to perk up my self-love life. It's like going out to a nice meal (with an employee discount) when you are not hungry. My friends' advice is echoing in my head saying, "This is the perfect time to get a new vibrator—you've got the time, and only yourself to please." But I'm sad and hurt—and sadness, for me, does not beget horniness.

So I just kick around the hippest sex store in town, testing vibrators in my hand and feeling glum.

**My first vibrator was given to
me as a Hannukah present
when I was twenty-three. I
was a late bloomer to masturbating and hadn't started
(at least consciously) doing
it until college, so this wasn't
that odd.** Also, it was technically
a "back massager," but we all
know what it was meant to do.
The same friend gave me my
second vibrator (let's call her my
vibrator whisperer), which was a
full-fledged penis re-creation in
blue. Anyway, I eventually started
buying my own vibrators and am
now on my fourth or fifth. I have
figured out my relationship with
vibrators to a T, and I would say
it's a healthy one.

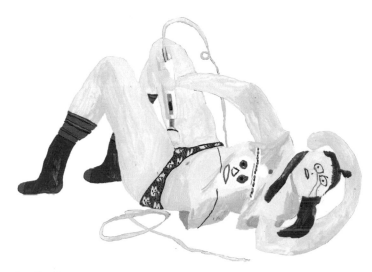

Tara Booth

Last year I was traveling with
my mom to Florida and it was the
first time we had been on a vacation without my dad or brother
in a long time. My mom and I are
very close, and she has always
freely talked to me about sex and
my body and encouraged me to
be open with her. When I was
younger and first felt a "tingle"
down there from watching a sex
scene in a movie, I didn't hesitate
to ask her what this was about,
and she didn't hesitate to be honest with me about it. We were
not a household of repression.

Anyway, it was winter in
Florida, and we somehow started
talking about masturbation. I
learned that my mother—my
sexually open mother, who had
been a Playboy waitress—had

never owned a vibrator! I was in
shock. How was this possible?
Yes, she was born in the early
1940s, but she had come of age
during the sexual revolution.

After I got over my shock, I
decided this had to be rectified.
So I googled where the closest
sex shop was to our Airbnb, and
lo and behold, just a few miles
away was a store that could
provide a possible solution to all
the sexual and kinky fantasies one
might have. My mom was super-
keen on my idea, and we drove
over. The clerk was unfazed by
a mother and daughter shopping
together. (I guess this is more
common than I thought.) We
looked around, laughing at the
various paraphernalia, and finally
asked the clerk to recommend
a simple-but-sure-thing vibrator. We didn't need the bunny
rabbit or the bullet or anything
fancy; we needed a three-speed
straight shot to the clitoris that

could get the job done, and we
found it. Before we left, I took
a picture of my mom holding it
and smiling, knowing I couldn't
post this on social media or show
it to my friends. It was our special
moment captured in time.

The vibrator was $40 and it
was a present from me to my
seventy-four-year-old mother,
which was more than I had ever
spent on my own vibrators. She
told me she was going to keep
it in her bedside table. When
I asked if she was going to tell
my dad, she scoffed: "No, why
would I do that? It doesn't have
anything to do with him!" That
answer is one of the many reasons I love my mom.

Every now and then since this
special day, I'll ask her if she's
using it, and she'll say, "Oh,
yeah!" with a big smile. And I can
proudly say that was $40 I don't
regret spending, and a shopping
expedition I won't ever forget.

A BRIEF HISTORY OF SEX TOYS

28,000 BC
SILT STONE DILDO
Eight-inch carved dildo discovered at Hohle Fels cave in Germany.

500
BEN WA BALL
Marble-size weighted ball that was inserted into the vagina to pleasure a man during intercourse.

1200
GOAT EYELID COCK RING
Made from goat eyelid with lashes intact for extra stimulation; used by Chinese nobility to increase fertility.

1869
THE MANIPULATOR
Steam-powered vibrator invented by Dr. George Taylor as a cure for "hysteria" in women. The engine was hidden in another room, and the dildo apparatus stuck out a hole in the wall.

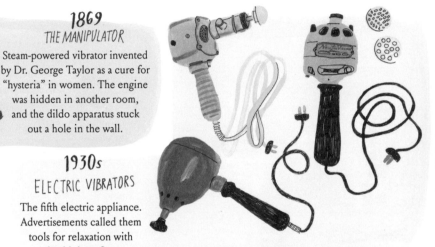

1930s
ELECTRIC VIBRATORS
The fifth electric appliance. Advertisements called them tools for relaxation with health benefits.

1960s
STRAP-ON DILDOS
The first strap-ons were designed by ventriloquist Ted Marche for impotent men.

1960s
HITACHI MAGIC WAND
Launched during the rise of the sex-positive movement, it became a bestseller and was used to teach masturbation.

1970s SILICONE DILDOS
Gosnell Duncan had an accident and became paralyzed and unable to have an erection. He designed his own silicone dildos in his basement. Eventually he partnered with the first sex toy shops, Eve's Garden and Good Vibrations, and created the first non-phallic dildos.

1984
THE RABBIT
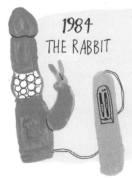
A dual-action vibrator that looks like a rabbit to adhere to Japan's "obscenity" laws. Rotating pearls in the shaft add more stimulation. This toy was popularized on *Sex and the City*.

Answering the Question

by JIZ LEE

There's a question everyone working in porn will be asked at least once in their career: "How did you get into porn?"

Depending on who's asking it, the question takes different forms. While it can be innocent in tone, it often assumes biased implications. Some common ones: that working in porn is not a real job and therefore a novelty (as if porn workers are not real people with lived experiences outside the contained fantasy of your computer screen); that the performer doesn't fit what you think of when you imagine a porn star, being either "too pretty" or "not pretty enough" (spoiler: sex workers come in all kinds); that the decision to get into porn is so outlandish from any other kind of job (and one so rife with stigma) that the career choice is foolish—if it was even a choice at all.

It is for the reasons above that this question is one I've been loathe to answer. Yet when I think back on all the times I've encountered it, I realize that I've answered it differently. And that my responses actually reveal a great deal about my intentions. I've continually asked myself this very question over the years I've worked in the industry. The "dialogue" goes something like this:

How did you get into porn? (2005)

I got lucky! I happened to be at the right place at the right time, being invited to perform in a scene by someone who wound up being my partner in love and art for many years. I would later joke that *Wanna do a porn scene with me?* is the perfect pickup line.

A recent transplant from Maui, Hawai'i, to Oakland, California, I first ventured out on my own far away from home—and in full bloom. I was discovering myself and coming out in multiplicities: as queer, as gender nonbinary, as polyamorous, and as a young adult hungry for sexual information and experiences. My sex education growing up in a small town was woefully inadequate, but San Francisco's LGBTQ+ mecca provided plenty of opportunities for personal growth through sex-ed classes, polyamorous workshops, play parties, and porn screenings.

Of course, I had stumbled across pornography as a teenager. Late at night, one of the TV channels became scrambled, revealing a distortion of naked blond bodies and the occasional nipple close-up. I later learned this soft-core pornography was called "Skinamax." However, the fact that it was censored might have been the only thing exciting about it. Of the other rare glimpses of "sexy" adults I saw, it just didn't seem like anything I could relate to. Not until I was in my twenties—sitting in a small theater in the Mission District, watching a screening of queer and trans sex—did I finally find it. What I saw was less about what one looked like than about who one *was*. I saw a reflection of myself and my community with all kinds of bodies having sex that was messy with raw emotion and defiant jubilance, and I knew immediately that I wanted to be on that screen.

My opportunity came in 2005, when I replied an enthusiastic *yes* to the pickup line that would catapult me deep into a summer of lust along with my first porn scene, in Shine Louise Houston's debut adult film, *The Crash Pad*. In the time between agreeing to the shoot and the production date, we had skyrocketed into a full-blown relationship with limerence on blast. The two of us awoke early that morning to head to the set. I was nervous only up until the cameras started rolling. On set, the quiet and shy side of my personality fades away and a confident, commanding performer shines. I kept present and connected to my partner, as I demonstrated my athleticism and sexual abilities. The shoot was collaborative and sweaty, and as I hopped up on the couch to hover over her face for my final, explosive cum shot, I knew I'd found my calling. It was an experience that cemented my passions and emotions around sharing sex on camera, and the film's release inspired a new wave of queer-made adult movies. The rest, as they say, is porn history.

How did *you* get into porn? (2010)

"You don't look like a typical porn star" is a statement I hear almost as often as the question that follows it. Because I live far from LA's porn valley and have an androgynous appearance (one director said I "wasn't porn pretty," comments call me "mannish," and an adult award show red-carpet host brushed me off as "too alternative"), projects in which I am a good fit are rare.

The majority of my work has existed within queer and trans indie adult-film projects that welcome my gender expression as an essential part of what makes me sexy. I've dabbled in "mainstream porn" where I could—to varying results. But I would argue that I landed on directors' radar in the first place precisely because I was so different.

Sometimes I approached performing for a company as being a "gateway queer"—that is, opening the doors to that company hiring other trans and nonbinary performers. However, I found that most directors were not so open-minded. A few even lied about how I would be presented. For example, one director lavished me with praise, professing how much he admired me as a leader in the nonbinary community. I thanked him, and we talked about how my scenes would be placed not within his lesbian titles, but in a new line that didn't misgender me. I shouldn't have been surprised when they went straight into his girl-on-girl line, with all the usual marketing.

While it was always a disappointment, I accepted the misgendering, thinking that at least my appearance might provide an androgynous, gender-nonconforming option for those who didn't know it was possible—that viewers might see me and know it's okay to be who they are, too. If they could then seek me out, it was still a positive outcome.

And it has blown me away when I get that feedback from fans. I've received emails, letters, and cards from people who found my work affirming. The other day on my commute into San Francisco, for example, someone slipped me a note and smiled as they exited the train. I waited until we rolled away from the station platform to open it:

Dear Mx Lee, I admire your work. It has helped me be more comfortable in my own body. Thank you.

What most people may not realize is that these messages mean just as much to me; they validate my own experience in sharing myself.

Any misdirected comment about me being ugly or not feminine enough only solidifies to me the need for more diversity regarding who gets to be seen as sexy. These messages confirm my belief, and they mean so much to receive. It is not a one-sided compliment. We are mirrors to each other—proof that we are visible, that we exist, that we are deserving of a happy and healthy sexuality in which we *thrive*.

How did you get *into* porn? (2015)

About ten years into the business, I found myself with a full-time porn day job, working behind the scenes with Shine Louise Houston at the company where I started. I'd finally secured an LLC and was on the way to trademarking my name. Finally, porn no longer felt like a side gig. Ten years in, I was in the thick of it and still finding ways to grow.

By now, porn was not only personal, it was political. I found myself taking on the role of advocate. Being in porn means fighting for it—and fighting for sex-worker rights at large.

How did you get into *porn*? (2020)

When I did my first film, I didn't feel like a porn performer.

I was headfirst in love, doing a scene with my partner, feeling nervous and curious to see what it would be like. Fast-forward fifteen years and I'm in it for life.

I'm a bigger champion of the porn industry than ever. My role now exists primarily as a facilitator and mentor behind the scenes. I strive to support emerging and indie filmmakers, helping them understand the ins and outs of the industry.

I continue to perform in porn, appearing in new films each year, approaching each project as it comes to see how I can bring my passion to the film and best represent myself and performers like me.

One of the most recent films I appeared in is a docu-porn that profiles actress Kali Sudhra as she travels to Germany to attend Pornfilmfestival Berlin. Woven into her story are interviews with festivalgoers from around the world—a vibrant backdrop of sex workers and artists who share a common vision of sexual expression and acceptance. The camera observes as Kali and I prepare for our scene, discussing our ideas with its director. Our highly stylized shoot blends athleticism, bondage, and Marlene Dietrich–inspired fashion, but the *cinema verité* depiction of its process and community reveals the profound importance of this work. I watch and rejoice in the spirit of the festival and its passionate creators who share our mission. I witness myself, eyes locked with Kali's, present for every minute of it. We kiss and we come and we talk and we laugh. We work, we communicate, we respect. As rare as it is to be a nonbinary performer in this industry—to watch myself on-screen and work with people who see me—I feel a sense of pride in being recognized and loved for who I am. It is absolutely a gift.

Is my story unique? The sex trade is vast, the adult-film industry wide and varied. Stories that are good and bad exist, though the media will want to focus on the worst outcomes as moral punishment. Stigma and shame will lead many to believe that nothing good can come from having sex on camera. But the truth is that you will find any story you want if you look hard enough. And this is mine.

How did I get into porn? With passion and perseverance. After all these years, I still believe it was the best decision I've ever made.

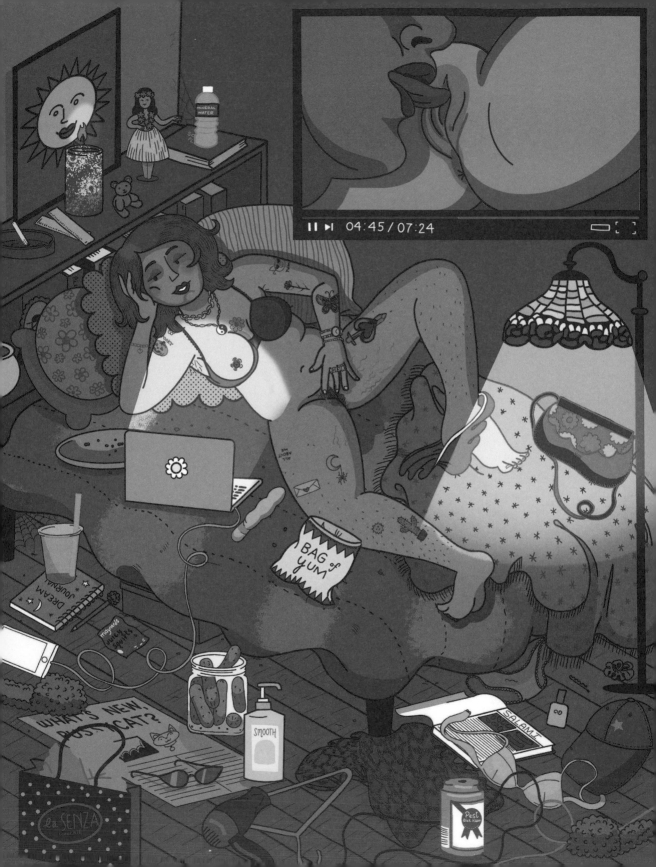

PORN

JULIA The first porn I ever saw was a woman giving head to a horse. A kid in my class showed a whole bunch of us. It was when the internet first came out.

SHAINA That's intense for a first porn experience. Mine was much more chill: it was some kind of soft-core porn on cable TV—I remember watching it with my friend and her brother in their TV room. Afterward I was like, *So* that's *what people are doing!*

I like bondage porn. I like rough-sex porn. It can't be too fake-looking, like big fake titties or too much makeup. **I like my porn people to be natural-looking.** I used to just watch white people—I'm Afro-Latina, but I would just watch white porn. Now, though, I watch black porn. But it has to feel real. Like it can't be like they're trying really hard to be black.

When I first looked at porn, twelve or thirteen years old, it was easier to find really hard-core stuff. Early on, I saw something I can't unsee: it was a woman giving a pig fellatio. **That image is one I can't forget.**

I watch porn with my boyfriend sometimes. We search for "threesomes" and "interracial" porn. He's black too, but I prefer watching interracial sex—I don't know why. Also "BBC"—Big Black Cock.

And I sometimes watch lesbian porn. I think of myself as bisexual, and he knows and is cool with it. He's very stingy with me, so we haven't done threesomes yet. But I'm interested.

I'm not really into porn or strip clubs. **You get all hot, but then nobody's there but you.**

Seeing a *Playboy* was a big deal, but there was no insertion it was just a naked woman. Then I saw my first VHS. It was two people, a man and a woman with a big bush, and they were doing missionary. It wasn't much to see. I didn't see any ridiculous shit until I was eighteen, luckily. That was scat porn. **My friend's roommate had that porn, and I could not believe it when I saw it. I wish I could unsee it.**

I was born in 1978. It was a magical time. You just had these snippets of a *Playboy* or a VHS tape. The true scarring didn't happen until the internet came around. Very quickly I learned not to google a lot of things. Too bad eleven-year-olds are having to do that now.

I work on a boat. We are
out on the Mississippi River.
I work twenty-eight days,
then home fourteen days. It's
just guys. I masturbate every
two days probably. I use porn.
It depends on the day, what I
look for. You want a bigger
woman sometimes, an Asian
woman another time. You're
gone so long on the boat that
when you get home, you just
want anybody. I'm just
being honest.

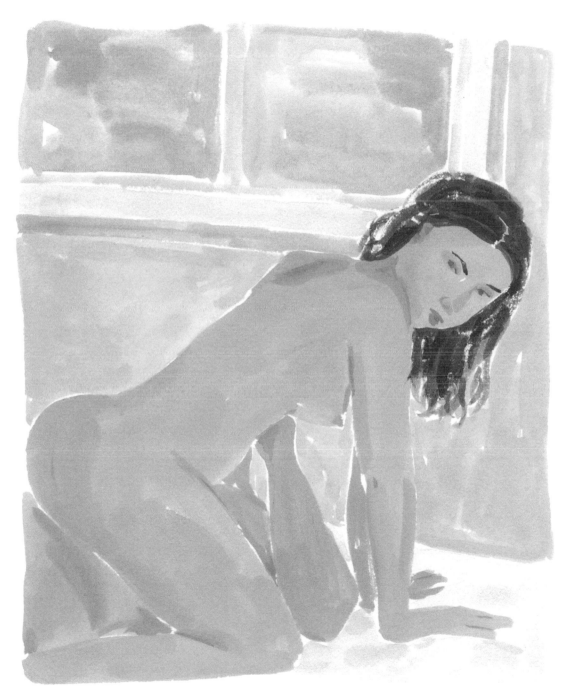

Leah Goren

I remember the first time I realized that I am definitely not straight, and that I definitely am attracted to guys. Whenever I hear other people's stories, it's always something along the lines of "I saw this movie with this actor and got a crush on him" or "I met this classmate and I realized I wanted to be with him," or the one we've all heard: "I've just known ever since I was a child." But none of those apply to me.

When I was thirteen and had just entered puberty, I started looking at pornography. I was too afraid to use a computer, because my parents had talked about putting parental locks on it that might track which sites I went on, and I didn't want my parents to find that out (they were both middle-aged conservative Christians). So I ended up looking at porn via the browser on my Nintendo DSi. Because of this I could only look at images, so naturally I realized that "furry porn" is a thing after a short amount of time. This is what led me down the rabbit hole, no pun intended, to understanding my sexuality, and it all happened one night when I was fourteen.

I was looking up furry porn on my DSi one night when I saw this one gay image. I had seen it before—the search terms I used weren't exactly creative or varied—but this time it awakened something inside me— something I didn't even know I had lying dormant. It was a drawing of two anthropomorphic dog-men having anal sex, with the bottom coming. When I saw that image this time, it caught my attention and I immediately wanted to be that bottom: I wanted to be with a guy sexually. I wanted someone to do that to me, and to make me feel like that.

Needless to say, I haven't really told anyone about this experience. It's kind of hard to say, "Ah yes, I discovered my sexuality through gay furry porn as a horny fourteen-year-old with only a DSi at his disposal."

In high school, I was the kid burning DVDs of porn and handing them out to my friends. **A lot of MILF porn—because they had huge tits and there was an aspect of nurturing.** Plus it was naughty. And there was this porn star Peter North, whose claim to fame was that he could shoot big loads. He had a secret diet to get a big load. I had a lot of his videos on the DVDs. And Seymore Butts's, too.

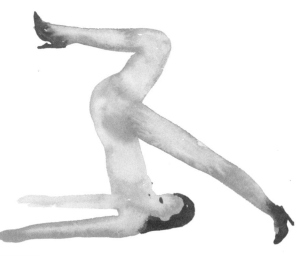

Ohni Lisle

One time my boyfriend and I taped ourselves during sex. We set up a minicam on the coffee table. In my mind I imagined myself looking way hotter. **But when I saw the video I was kind of grossed out.** It was in college and I misplaced that cassette somewhere.

I got a hard-on for erotica at an early age. I'd sneak looks at *Playboy* in a local convenience store, then gaze at issues circulated at Scout camps. By the time I reached high school in the 1970s, *Penthouse* became my porn of choice, along with the *Penthouse* letters—a carnival of astounding acts like threesomes and shaved cunts.

One summer day I used *Penthouse* to whack off three times, still my personal record. I couldn't do that now if you put a gun to my head, but Sofía Vergara next to my head...that might work.

After college I dabbled in *Swank* and *High Society,* but none inspired brand loyalty. Best-of-*Penthouse* collections in the '80s gave me the serious thrill. Bob Guccione's flushed, yearning women nestled in my libido with their Pre-Raphaelite languor and lingerie, the nipple stroking and lip licking.

Then I met my wife, but I was too hard-wired into the porn/masturbation cycle—that's not so easy to break. I'm ashamed to say that my wife got the full focus of my sexual energy only in the early years of our relationship (or the early *months*). Every relationship settles some after the first heat wave breaks, but ours settled more like the *Titanic*

on the Atlantic floor. Worse, we couldn't talk about fantasies or unmet expectations—until that day when she bitterly said she'd been faking her orgasms. In my heart I knew I'd shortchanged her, and I tried to change, but our sexual relationship only worsened as our marriage deteriorated. Her cougarish post-divorce vibe, with the short leather skirt, left me trembling when family matters brought us together. Her confidence declared she was more than ready to make up for lost time with tall, competent lovers.

Divorce freed me to indulge in the world of online porn. Well, why not? Saddled with debt and a small apartment, I was nobody's idea of a dating dreamboat. Sequentially, I subscribed to Abby Winters, Sapphic Erotica, Penthouse, X-Art, Hegre, and Morey Studio. Then I stopped, tired of it all. I contented myself with free porn, narrowing down to a handful of sites that looked the safest from viruses.

Even that shrank to a few porn genres and styles of photography, like the high gloss of Digital Desire and the shadowed, fetishy mood of the Life Erotic. **Ultimately, my own digital desires faded with my drooping level of testosterone and the realization that I had seen everything,**

discarded 99 percent of it, and was spinning my wheels over the same endless track. The five seconds of benefit didn't justify the half hour of monumental mental and physical effort. More than horniness, habit and loneliness pushed me along.

Anyway, the current look of porn bores me. I don't respond to thin nude models with pumped-up boobs splayed on cold tile floors under antiseptic lights. Tattoos and punk hairstyles are repulsive. *Penthouse*'s lush adoration of the female form became a '70s anachronism that only old guys like me still adore; erotica slumped into anatomy lessons. I can easily go for weeks without any interest in the flipbooks of familiar images. My time shifted to better uses (such as writing this).

The biggest winner: my long-term significant other. I no longer struggle with the exhaustion, semi-impotence, and stabbing headaches that helped wreck my marriage. The mental tumult mostly eased as the neural pathways cleared. I joke with my partner, "I've got a full head of steam tonight," not quite explaining myself. "It's been a couple of weeks, we're both all backed up." And that works for us.

The Fruit I Carry

by RACHEL EVANS

There is an alien growing inside me."

"No there isn't, Rach—I can hardly see it."

"First off, that's a lie. But second of all, even if you couldn't 'see' this five-inch bulge here"—I point at my belly, implicating their lies—"it's how I feel. I *feel* like there's an alien growing inside me."

My friend, nameless and faceless, nods in an attempt to understand. Nameless and faceless, because I've had this conversation with too many friends to count, and only nods, because I've felt this way for so long that all they can really do at this point is nod.

It's not a baby. The alien, that is. If it was a baby, it would be a zygote and then a peppercorn and then a blueberry and then a sweet potato and then a cantaloupe—week after week, it would graduate to a larger fruit until it reached the apex: the watermelon, a full-size baby, ready to be born. If it was a baby, it would grow and kick and probably make me uncomfortable and nauseous and in awe of my own body and then uncomfort-

able again, but at the end of forty weeks (or so), it would no longer be in me, it would be out in the world. If it was a baby, it would be a blessing, a brachah; it would be a dream, and a miracle.

Rather, instead, I have felt bloated and uncomfortable because of my glorious fibroid—my noncancerous tumor that was discovered when I was thirty. It was considered rather large for someone my age—so large that the ultrasound technician inappropriately gasped, did a double take, and asked, "How old are you again?"

For almost eight years my fibroid grew inside me, getting larger with each passing year—and, as I would find out from an MRI—partially collapsing my bladder. This MRI also revealed that my vagina is "unremarkable," which I found out is a good thing, but I take issue with these semantics. After almost forty years with my vagina, it is far from unremarkable (but that's for another essay, another time).

When I finally had good health insurance and my fibroid had grown to eleven centimeters (equivalent to a four-month-size fetus—a cantaloupe!), I had surgery to have it removed. After five hours in the operating room, the surgeon removed the fibroid laparoscopically (through my belly button, no less), and took out a cyst he found as well, because two for the price of one. Within just a few weeks I was beginning to rebuild my core and get my old body back; my energy was returning and I was living FF—Fibroid-Free!

And then a funny thing happened. I noticed that my innie belly button, which was still discolored and healing, had become an outie. A few days later, I realized my belly button was missing altogether. I searched and searched my stomach but could not find that cute little hole that once was. I now had a protrusion where it should have been.

Naturally, I went to the surgeon to ask him to find my belly button. Instead, he gave my new problem a name: *hernia*. Turns out my first surgery had inadvertently led to an "incisional hernia," and now another surgery was required to fix it. In the general vicinity of where there had once been a large mass, I now had a hole inside me where my intestine was pushing through, creating a very noticeable bulge in my belly. One alien had been removed, but a new one was gestating.

Obviously it's a crummy turn of luck when you finally fix a problem and the solution creates a new one. But the extra-special kick in the tuchus is that it's all happening around my abdomen. So much unwanted attention and negative growth in a part of me that really only wants one thing: a baby.

In the last year and a half, I have had three medical procedures all in the same neighborhood (of my body). Last year I froze my eggs, which required ten days of injecting my belly with hormones and then a retrieval of my healthy, now-younger eggs. This year brought a myomectomy (to get that long-lasting fibroid) and finally the hernia-repair surgery. Eggs have been removed, a fibroid has been suctioned, a hole has been patched up. My body has been stretched, prodded, probed, and punctured in the same place where my heart desires a healthy being to grow and emerge.

I carry around disappointment the size of a pineapple that this hasn't happened in my life yet—no partner, no union, no baby. And sometimes I wonder if this sadness I am holding has taken tangible form as the fibroid and hernia. I'm irrationally afraid that my melancholic emotions have warped inside me into real-life cells and tissue and weakened abdominal walls.

Ever since my seven eggs (a good number for a woman "my age"!) were retrieved from me and cryogenically frozen, I have thought of them often. I thank them for their youth and impermanent presence as a backup plan for me, and I diligently pay their rent on time twice a year. Before my fibroid surgery, I lit a candle and some incense and meditated to say goodbye to this thing that had lived within me for so many years. I know that sounds super hippie-dippie (and let's face it—it was), but I felt like even though it had

caused me discomfort and grief, it had also been with me through heartbreak, through adventure, through love and loss, through eight years of my life. I did not do that for the hernia. I had no attachment to that hole in my fascia. It was merely a hole.

My belly now bears five small scars and a newly built belly button. They form a maze of tiny imprints that lead nowhere, a road map of resilience.

Before my hernia surgery, I would often find myself unconsciously rubbing my stomach, slowly soothing my distended abdomen with repetitive circles. It was the same way that I rubbed my belly when it was bloated from all the shots, or when my fibroid was protruding. This specific rubbing has a name in the Lamaze community: *effleurage,* or the rhythmic and repeated stroking of the belly. It was an act of comfort, yet it also created a distance between myself and reality. Because at some point in the circular caressing, I forgot what part of myself I was comforting. And the outside world, which doesn't know what is or isn't in me, observed something else: they saw a pregnant woman speaking to her unborn baby.

And in the forgetting, and the smiles from strangers, this surgery-laden belly of mine transformed into an imagined hope. And then I wondered: What if these problems—these spaces filled with pain and discomfort—could magically transform into a future soul? What if all this time spent preparing and recovering could yield my greatest wish—a squealing, smiling baby? How do I rearrange my body and this energy, and focus the space in my middle into joy?

I don't know the answer, but I'll say it has not been easy. And so I paused the rubbing and placed my hand over the area where the belly button should have been, in tenderness and gratitude and hope, and I said a prayer of awe—for all my body can be capable of, and for all it can still want and find room for.

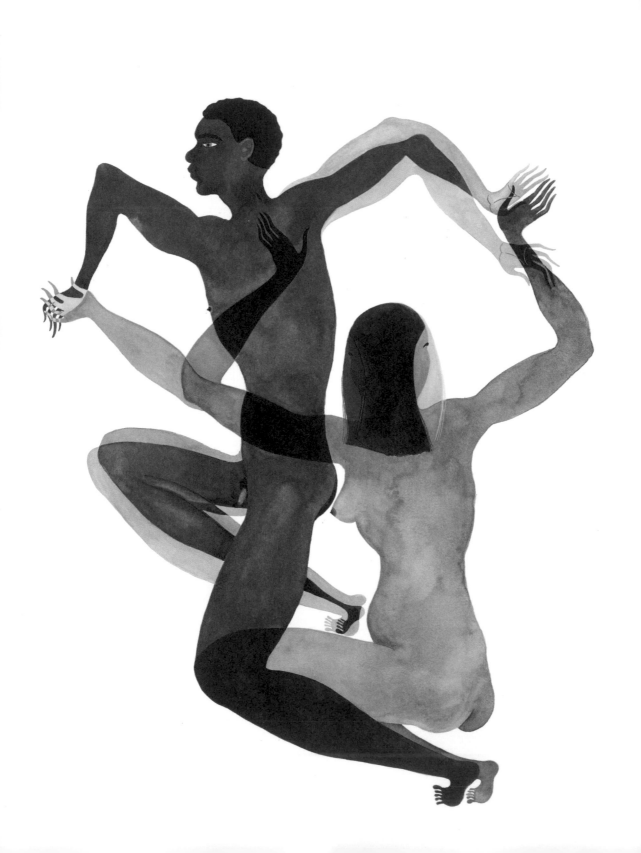

FERTILITY, PREGNANCY & MISCARRIAGE

SHAINA I had a really early miscarriage and it was so sad. And I felt exhausted from it for like two weeks.

JULIA I remember the day you told me. I didn't know what to do or say.

SHAINA It's hard to know what to say to someone. But when I had mine, I found out that so many of my friends and family have had them. We're simply not talking about them openly.

Growing up, I had the typical American East Coast sex ed in schools: *Don't have sex; you'll get pregnant immediately and ruin your life.*

So when I met my future husband at sixteen years old, we waited three years to have sex for the first time. **He was terrified I would get pregnant. I was terrified I would get pregnant.** But I didn't get pregnant, because I got on the pill. I was on the pill for ten years.

We went to college, got married, lived in three different states, built and lost careers, got a dog. Before I turned twenty-nine, I felt my biological clock start ticking. We had worked so hard to get to a good place in life. We waited a long time to feel stable—in our home, in our jobs, in our bank account, in our minds—but now I wanted a baby more than ever. More than anything, I wanted a baby with the man I love—the man who knew that getting me pregnant at seventeen would probably ruin my life.

So we ditched the birth control. I got off my non-pregnancy-safe antidepressant (a truly crappy experience). I charted my cycles. I peed on ovulation sticks. We had timed sex. We struggled with timed sex. I didn't get pregnant. We tried again and again and again. I'm still not pregnant.

Sex isn't fun anymore—it's like a job. I feel betrayed. Betrayed by the school system that said it was so easy to get pregnant. Betrayed by my body. Betrayed by being a responsible adult who waited until the right moment to build a family.

Balint Zsako

Something clicked in my mid-thirties, when I realized that all my hooking up had been fun but now I was ready to find "the one"—and I did. At the fine age of thirty-seven, I met my future husband. We wanted the same things out of life, had shared values, and he was very honest and kind.

And cute, too, but our sex life was only okay. He wasn't very experienced, and he had the smallest penis of anyone I'd ever been with. I hardly ever got off during sex. We got married when I was thirty-nine, and we started trying to get pregnant right away. Sex really wasn't fun anymore. I was checking my temperature, checking when I was ovulating, timing when we should try. Within a year, I was (miraculously) pregnant and gave birth when I was forty-one. But it was a long, hard labor: I had third-degree tearing, and my son was delivered with forceps. (For readers who don't know, fourth-degree tearing is when your perineum rips all the way to your anus. So mine was not *that* bad, but still it was traumatic. And if you've ever seen gynecological forceps, they're the size of metal spatulas you'd use on the grill.)

My son also had some complications at birth, so I was an emotional wreck as well. It took a long time for my body to physically heal, and when it did, it was definitely not the same. I had hard scar tissue in my vaginal opening; inserting even a tampon hurt. I was embarrassed to ask my doctor about it but finally brought it up. I talked to her about wanting to get pregnant again, so she recommended a fertility-friendly lube.

The problem?

My libido was shot. I didn't know if it was because I knew sex was still going to be uncomfortable and possibly painful, or if it was because I

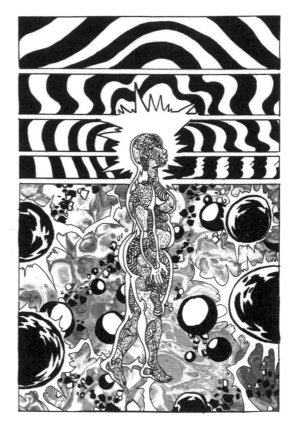

Sloane Leong

was in my early forties and starting to show signs of perimenopause. We finally went to see a fertility specialist, who said our best chance of getting pregnant with my eggs and his sperm was via IUI, or intrauterine insemination. (We weren't good candidates for in vitro fertilization because at forty-four I was already too old.) We were still supposed to try during times of ovulation, but between going to acupuncture to increase my egg production and taking supplements and tracking when I was ovulating and going for vaginal ultrasounds to check my follicle, doing an injection to release the egg at the right time, and dealing with a kid with sleep issues—to say nothing of work and life stress—sex was unappealing. I never did get pregnant again.

I have no desire for sex with my husband, but I do enjoy masturbating. **I just regret not talking to my doctor earlier about my fertility.**

I spent three years trying to get pregnant and lost two of them — it's really difficult. As lesbians, I still say, "She got me pregnant." We had a donor who gave us a cup of sperm, and then I used a syringe and did it myself. We had already done all the doctor shit; this was our last-ditch effort, and it worked.

About three years after our second child was born, my wife started asking if I wanted to have another. I was skeptical, but eventually I came around—it would be worth that sleepless first year to have more love and joy for the rest of our lives. But it wasn't working. We were in the latter half of our thirties when our oldest was born, and we had rounded forty by now. We weren't terribly surprised, and the trying was fun, so we just kept trying—everywhere!

Each month when my wife was about to ovulate, she'd get super turned on, as nature surely intended. For the most part we took care of business after the kids were in bed, but once in a while we'd have to put them in front of a (loud) movie or something in the middle of the day while we closed our door.

One time we were canoe camping on a tiny island in the middle of a lake. We were packing up lunch when she gave me that look. There was no TV to turn on for the kids, but it was ovulation time and we were feeling lucky about this try.

We set the kids up with some activity or other and told them we had to fuss with the food pack to make sure no bears visited our camp later on. We crossed our fingers and slipped into the woods, where we'd hung our food pack in a tree.

Problem #1: We looked around at all the sticks and pine needles and sharp rocks. No way were we rolling around on the ground. Instead, my wife dropped her shorts and pulled me to her, standing against the closest tree. If you've ever tried sex while standing in the woods hoping your children don't find you, you know what I'm talking about. Aim was a bit of a challenge, but we got things working eventually.

Problem #2: I'm a lot taller than my wife is, and even though she stood on slightly higher ground, I ended up doing a partial squatthrust to get everything aligned. This was fine at first, but given the circumstances (having sex while standing in the woods while hoping our children wouldn't find us) it was taking me some time to "get there." My legs were burning with muscle fatigue, and I was starting to sweat. A lot.

Problem #3: Perhaps you already know this, but increased physical activity makes your body emit more carbon dioxide. And you may know this, too, but certain forest dwellers are attracted by carbon dioxide. No, not bears; mosquitoes.

So there we were, having sex while standing in the woods and hoping our children wouldn't find us, burning with muscle fatigue, sweating, and swatting at our most intimate areas as I tried to achieve an orgasm.

I will tell you now that I did not develop any pain-related kinks in the woods that day. And that I did find it difficult to scratch discreetly for a week or two afterward. And yes, though I nearly passed out from muscle fatigue and dehydration, definitely gave up hope, and had to stretch my aching quads for three days in the aftermath, I did finally succeed in achieving an orgasm while having sex while standing in the woods and hoping our children wouldn't find us, burning with muscle fatigue, sweating, and swatting at my most intimate areas.

And I will tell you that three years and six miscarriages later, our new daughter is four weeks old.

When I was nursing, I didn't want to have sex at all; I was totally over-touched. **I had my baby attached to me all the time.** My husband was a little bit frustrated about that. We were both concerned that we were never going to have sex again. But once I stopped nursing, my sex drive returned.

Since having kids, of course, we don't have as much sex as we used to because we are always tired. But I think we still have a very healthy sex life.

I've had twenty-nine miscarriages (my uterus is flipped and inverted), so having my kid was a miracle. **I was told I couldn't have kids when I went to get birth control in junior high.** I went to several different doctors; they all told me the same thing.

I always had very early miscarriages. I knew, so it wasn't sad. Then, when I finally did get pregnant, I didn't know. I'd never had regular periods, so when I went to the hospital in severe pain and they told me "You're in labor," I was like, "What the fuck?!"

I was in labor for two days. They spread my hips too wide, and now I have issues. And my uterus is still flipped and inverted. But my son was born seven pounds, twelve ounces, and I love him to death.

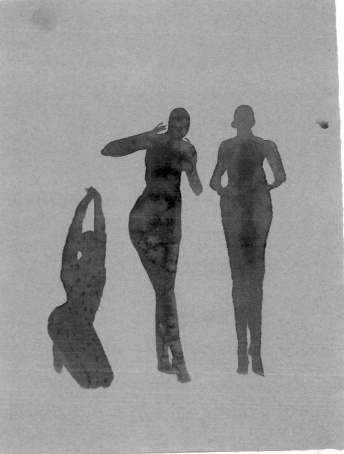

Chioma Ebinama

My friend got pregnant quickly and had a box of leftover ovulation strips. When she found out we were going to try to get pregnant, she mailed them to me with a note: "Good luck!" I excitedly woke up every morning and peed on the ovulation strip, waiting to see the smiley face. When it appeared I would jump back in bed and rip my clothes off, whispering "It's time!" to my husband.

He was horrified.

We had obligatory sex—maybe the worst, dullest sex we'd ever had. I started to be more subtle, using the strips secretly and then just trying to be sexier when I saw the smiley face—wearing tank tops that let my nipples point out, shaving my legs.

He saw through it.

We were on two separate teams, and all the spontaneity of just feeling it, and doing it, was gone. Ultimately we gave up the strips and conceived at a music festival—drunk, happy, and blissfully unaware of the egg traveling down my fallopian tube.

When my husband and I decided to conceive our first child, we had just moved back to the place where we were the happiest, as individuals and as a couple. It was where we wanted to raise our future tiny human. We had no family (ergo no drama or pressure), and all our friends from graduate school were there. We rented an overpriced home in a hip neighborhood and were still in a cloud of romance ten years after we met. It was joyous. It felt magical and serene.

Now here we are four years later with a three-year-old, back on the coast closer to our respective families. He works twelve-hour days at a physically demanding job; thanks to the outrageous price of childcare and preschool, I just quit mine to stay at home with our child. We coast financially. We want a sibling for our little one and a baby to love, despite the depressing worldwide news (which we try to counteract with friendliness, attempted minimalism, and homemaking at its best in the world of suburbia and budgets).

These are not grounds for the intimate, panting-worthy, *oh my god I'm so in love with you* sexy kind of sex. At ten o'clock—when the dishes are (possibly)

Jason Adam Katzenstein

"Emotionally, I'm leaving you. Physically, I pretty much need to stay right here."

done, the dog still needs to be walked, you have to pick up thirty items from each room, and your partner is already asleep as you remember you need to order contacts—you don't want to bother to try the sexy dance. Your naked body is so familiar to your partner in nonsexual ways that they don't acknowledge it when it's there.

Let's be honest: no matter how many years of marriage you have on you, this is emotionally painful. It hurts. You want him to want you, but you know he doesn't. He resents you for

asking for help with mundane things that he doesn't naturally do and loses that attraction. Conceiving the second child feels like the 1,487th ride on the Ferris wheel. You remember what the first thrilling time around felt like in your throat, and your heart skips a beat—only to find yourself with sticky, uncomfortable, cotton-candy hands, dirty laundry to deal with, and that thrill ride a memory retrievable only by seeing the other people in line who have yet to ride the wheel. Hey, let's do it one more time before I fall asleep, eh?

Today I had an ultrasound—the kind on your belly. I realized that, possibly, I will not have another intrauterine ultrasound for the rest of my life. Those are the kind where the probe is placed in your vagina. I had the first one seven years ago, at my gynecologist's office. I was getting tested for infertility. I had to do this step first, then my husband could come in for semen testing. That day, the sonographer squirted gel on my belly and ran an ultrasound wand across it to check out my ovaries—no cysts.

Then she said, "Did the doctor tell you we have to do the other kind as well?"

I said, "No, she didn't."

I knew about intrauterine ultrasounds only because they were in the news; women seeking abortions were being forced to have them in some states. Afterward, I went to my car and sobbed. The phrase *medical rape* did cross my mind. Had I really consented?

Today I'm on miscarriage watch for my sixth pregnancy. I'm ten weeks along, which is pretty good, but I've had sporadic bleeding from a small hemorrhage for the past few weeks. I have one daughter. She survived a hemorrhage, so I'm cautiously optimistic this one will stick too. If so, our reproductive journey will be complete. Life can move forward.

My other four pregnancies resulted in miscarriage before nine weeks. None of those pregnancies were created through sex. All required a medical team, probes, labs, and science. **We had plenty of sex over the years to achieve pregnancy, but it grew more demoralizing with each month, and then with each year, until it became borderline traumatic to try.**

Last week, my OB did a transvaginal ultrasound. During it, for a quick flash, I remembered that I will enjoy sex again. Lust and desire will return. I will be able to relax my body. I will welcome my husband's touch again. I could remember it.

I'm guessing I've had at least one hundred transvaginal ultrasounds over seven years, two insemination cycles, three IVF egg retrievals, and eight embryo-transfer cycles. Our daughter is lucky embryo No. 7.

This past month, my OB offered me weekly heartbeat checks to calm my nerves about a miscarriage. He was apologetic that the first few ultrasounds had to be intrauterine so he could do measurements and peek at the hemorrhage. Plus my uterus tilts backward; that's unrelated to my infertility, but it makes it harder to see a fetus from one's stomach. As he apologized, I coolly joked that I'd had a hundred of them before. He didn't laugh. His empathy made me want to cry.

Most of the women who did my other uterine probes were kind as well. Some were even apologetic (though others jammed the probe in with less warning and care). I saw one sonographer over several years, and we developed a special relationship. She worked at our first IVF clinic, where treatment resulted in my first two miscarriages (one ectopic—a pregnancy lodged in my fallopian tube). Soon after, we both left for a better clinic. I got a message to her when my daughter was finally born, after the first four years of trying. She bought me clothes for the baby to wear.

Sometime next year, I hope, my vagina will be mine again. I won't have to share it with a rotating cast of medical professionals. It will be of service to me again for pleasure, not grief. And sex will be for fun.

THINGS YOU MIGHT NOT KNOW ABOUT MISCARRIAGE BY JULIA WERTZ
(TRIGGER WARNING: GALLOWS HUMOR)

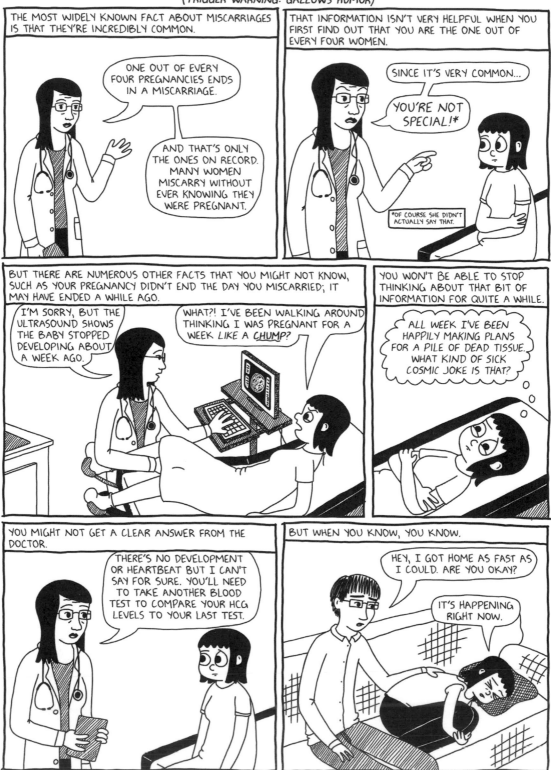

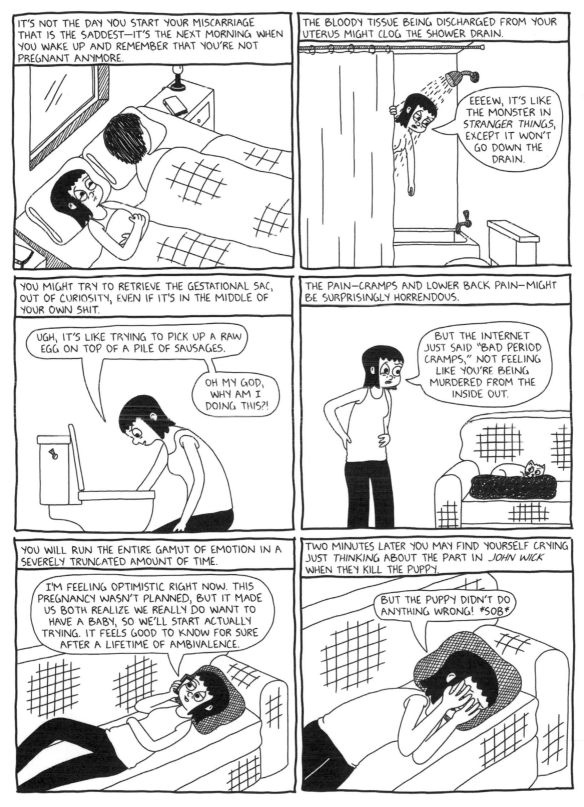

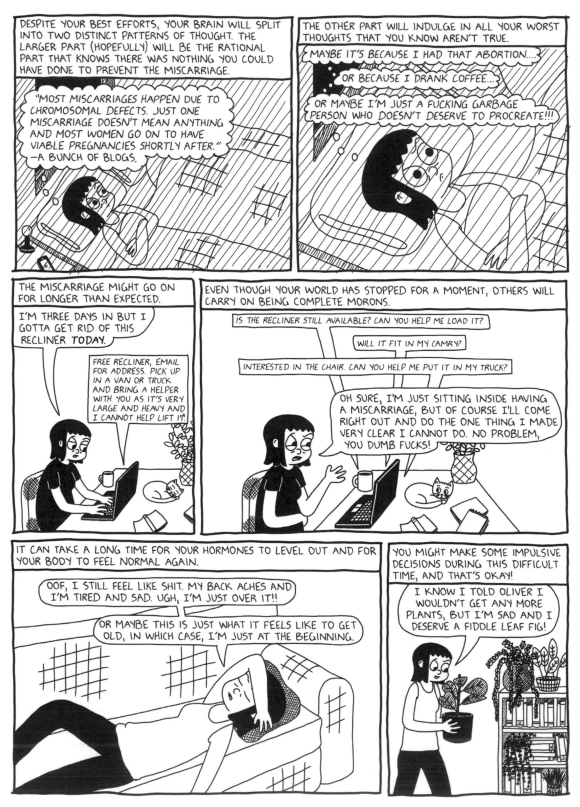

DESPITE YOUR BEST EFFORTS, YOUR BRAIN WILL SPLIT INTO TWO DISTINCT PATTERNS OF THOUGHT. THE LARGER PART (HOPEFULLY) WILL BE THE RATIONAL PART THAT KNOWS THERE WAS NOTHING YOU COULD HAVE DONE TO PREVENT THE MISCARRIAGE.

"MOST MISCARRIAGES HAPPEN DUE TO CHROMOSOMAL DEFECTS. JUST ONE MISCARRIAGE DOESN'T MEAN ANYTHING AND MOST WOMEN GO ON TO HAVE VIABLE PREGNANCIES SHORTLY AFTER." —A BUNCH OF BLOGS.

THE OTHER PART WILL INDULGE IN ALL YOUR WORST THOUGHTS THAT YOU KNOW AREN'T TRUE.

MAYBE IT'S BECAUSE I HAD THAT ABORTION....

OR BECAUSE I DRANK COFFEE....

OR MAYBE I'M JUST A FUCKING GARBAGE PERSON WHO DOESN'T DESERVE TO PROCREATE!!!

THE MISCARRIAGE MIGHT GO ON FOR LONGER THAN EXPECTED.

I'M THREE DAYS IN BUT I GOTTA GET RID OF THIS RECLINER TODAY.

FREE RECLINER, EMAIL FOR ADDRESS. PICK UP IN A VAN OR TRUCK AND BRING A HELPER WITH YOU AS IT'S VERY LARGE AND HEAVY AND I CANNOT HELP LIFT IT.

EVEN THOUGH YOUR WORLD HAS STOPPED FOR A MOMENT, OTHERS WILL CARRY ON BEING COMPLETE MORONS.

IS THE RECLINER STILL AVAILABLE? CAN YOU HELP ME LOAD IT?

WILL IT FIT IN MY CAMRY?

INTERESTED IN THE CHAIR. CAN YOU HELP ME PUT IT IN MY TRUCK?

OH SURE, I'M JUST SITTING INSIDE HAVING A MISCARRIAGE, BUT OF COURSE I'LL COME RIGHT OUT AND DO THE ONE THING I MADE VERY CLEAR I CANNOT DO. NO PROBLEM, YOU DUMB FUCKS!

IT CAN TAKE A LONG TIME FOR YOUR HORMONES TO LEVEL OUT AND FOR YOUR BODY TO FEEL NORMAL AGAIN.

OOF, I STILL FEEL LIKE SHIT. MY BACK ACHES AND I'M TIRED AND SAD. UGH, I'M JUST OVER IT!!

OR MAYBE THIS IS JUST WHAT IT FEELS LIKE TO GET OLD, IN WHICH CASE, I'M JUST AT THE BEGINNING.

YOU MIGHT MAKE SOME IMPULSIVE DECISIONS DURING THIS DIFFICULT TIME, AND THAT'S OKAY!

I KNOW I TOLD OLIVER I WOULDN'T GET ANY MORE PLANTS, BUT I'M SAD AND I DESERVE A FIDDLE LEAF FIG!

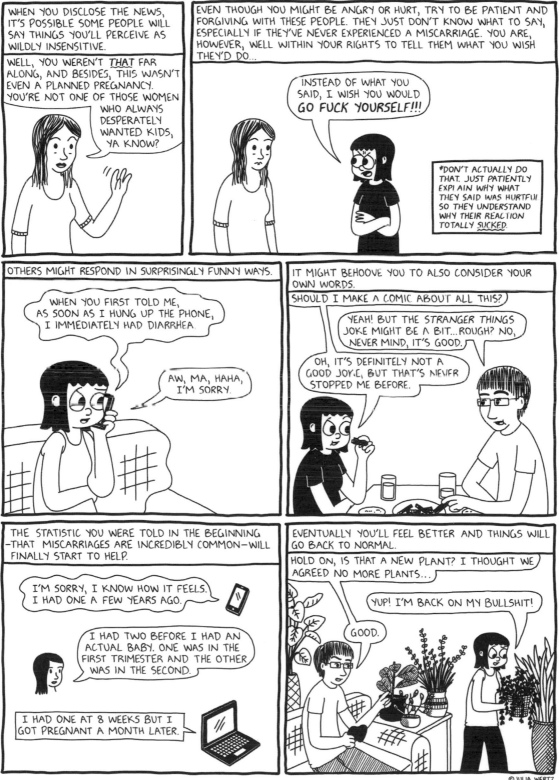

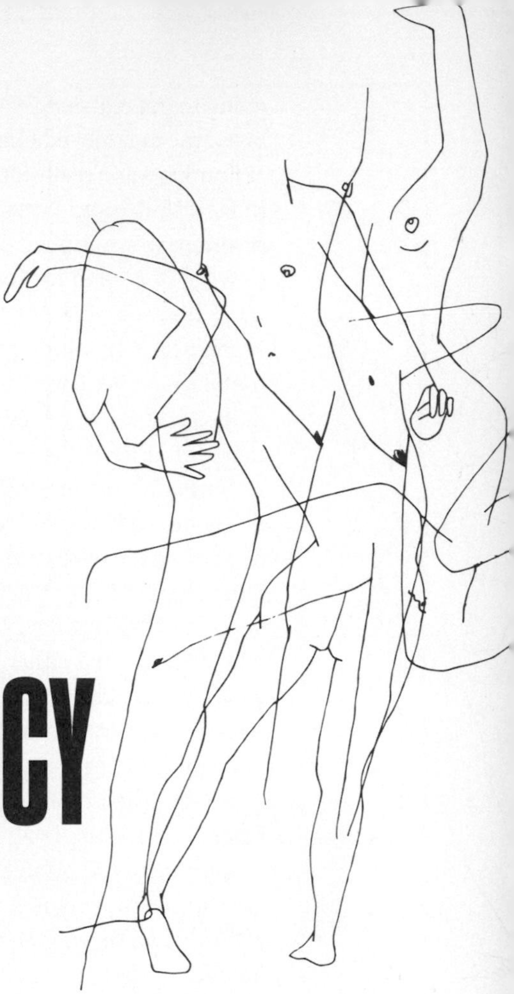

As Told To

TEEN PREGNANCY

ANONYMOUS

When I was sixteen, a junior in high school, I had a boyfriend, Frankie. I was on the cheering squad, and he was on the football team. I'm Jewish, and he was Italian. That was many years ago, in 1959, when Jewish girls were not supposed to date Italian guys. We used to fool around after we had known each other just a few months. Not right away, because in those days it was forbidden.

The forbidden part made it a little bit more exciting. If I had to go someplace, I would have a Jewish guy come pick me up and then, once outside, go and meet Frankie. We became a couple and spent every afternoon together. I would not tell my mom the truth because I was afraid I would hurt her.

My senior year of high school, Frankie and I started fooling around more. I started cutting school to fool around in my apartment after my mom and dad had left for work. We started doing some heavy stuff and eventually we started to make love. Back then, we were never taught about protection. The only thing my mom said when I first got my menstrual period was "Never let a boy touch you until you're married." But we were going to get married. We talked about it. I felt this sex thing was love: he loved me and I loved him.

Frankie was a really nice guy. He was going to go to art school—a college in New York—and I was going to a liberal arts college upstate. Over the summer, we continued our sexual relationship. My mom had gone away to work at a hotel for the summer and my father would go visit her on the weekends, so we had the place to ourselves. We never thought about protection. One time he took me to college, and we stayed overnight at a motel room. We used to have sex wherever we could—outside, on a rock or in the playground, or secretly in my apartment. But that night it was more intense because we had a proper bed.

At seventeen, I started college. All of a sudden my breasts hurt, I didn't feel good, and I was nauseous. I also didn't get my period for a while. I confided in a good girlfriend of mine, Dottie—we had grown up together—and Dottie said, "Let's go downtown and see if there's a doctor. Nobody will know us." We had never been to a gynecologist in our whole lives. None of my friends had either. So we went to New York City during Christmas vacation—Dottie and I, and Frankie came with us too. I went into a drugstore and got into a phone booth and looked up in the Yellow Pages the name of a doctor that was by Central Park. The first one I came to—going down the list at the beginning of the phone book—was a Dr. Armstrong. I called and said, "I'm here in New York City, home from college. I need to see a doctor and I need to have a rabbit test taken." (That's what they used to call the pregnancy test.)

I walk into the doctor's office. It's a big, beautiful office, and he's sitting behind his desk. I told Dr. Armstrong, "I'd like to have a rabbit test taken to find out if I'm pregnant."

He said, "How old are you?"

"I'm seventeen," I said. "I'm gonna be eighteen."

He asked me a bunch of questions, like, "Do your mother and father know?"

I said, "No, they don't. I just came here to find out if I am."

He said to me, "Okay, go over there and sit on the sofa."

I remember I was wearing a pleated skirt. He said, "Lean back." I lay down. He picked up my skirt and he pulled down my underpants. "Okay," he said, "now open your legs and just look at me."

He put his finger and hand in me and started feeling around inside me.

"I don't think you're pregnant," he said. "If you were, you'd have a certain kind of red ring around your vagina, and you don't have that."

I said, "Oh, great!"

He said, "But I'm gonna send you to my friend, who can do a rabbit test. Go to this laboratory." And he gave me the name and phone number.

I paid him and left, and I didn't think of it as anything. Now when I think back, I think, *How stupid could I have been?!* Years later I looked up that doctor again, and guess what his profession was? He was a psychiatrist—how about that?

It took a few days to get the rabbit test done, and they called Dottie with the results. She calls me and tells me, "You're pregnant." I was so ashamed. Abortion was illegal. It wasn't even an option that crossed my mind. I had to go tell my mother and father that I was four months pregnant!

My mom said, "Oh my, what are we going to do?" And my father walked the floor and was crying.

My mother never cursed—never even said *hell*—so this was the first time I'd ever heard her say a bad word. "I raised you to be a good girl, and now you're gonna have a shegetz bastard!"

And I said, "Mommy, Frankie and I want to get married. We love each other. We want to have a baby."

Meanwhile Frankie had already told his parents, and his dad said to him, "You're not getting married until I say you're getting married."

My mom called in a rabbi she knew, and the rabbi said to me, "You know you can't keep this baby. You can't marry him."

I felt I had to do whatever they told me to do. They wanted me to give the baby up for adoption, and the rabbi said he knew a female doctor in Pennsylvania who took in girls who were "wayward" and delivered their babies. I was told not to tell anyone about this. Everyone thought I was away at college. My sister didn't know, my brother didn't know. We lied to everyone.

My cousin Eli was my father's lawyer, so my parents went to Eli and told him what had happened. Eli and his wife, Cindy, had just gotten married, and she was pregnant herself. Eli and Cindy said I could come stay with them until the Pennsylvania doctor could take me. So I went to Eli and Cindy's apartment to hide out. They were so happy about the baby they would soon have, and here I was pregnant, waiting to go to a doctor to give up my baby. One time, a cousin of ours came to visit Eli. Nobody was supposed to know I was there, so I had to hide in the closet for two hours.

When it was time to go to the doctor, they had me leave in the middle of the night. I was sent to Penn Station with a little suitcase by myself to head to Pennsylvania. When I got to the train station in Pennsylvania someone was supposed to meet me, but they never showed up. All I had was an address on a piece of paper. I called a cab and it let me out at a big, beautiful house.

An old woman came to the door with, I swear, a kerosene lamp. She says, "I'm Dr. Cranbrook. It's nice to meet you." She said, "This is my office entrance, but we live in the back of the house." She said, "Don't be afraid that it's so dark—this is how it is at night."

She took me to a bedroom. It was very old-fashioned—a four-poster bed, with a book on the bedside table: *Painless Childbirth.* There was no lock on the door. I got into bed and thought, *I just have to deal with this.* Then

I thought about the book on the table. I didn't even know that childbirth could be *painful*!

Sitting at the kitchen table in the morning, Dr. Cranbrook said, "Don't worry. Whatever you want you can have here. I'm going to take good care of you." She taught me how to do the *New York Times* crossword puzzle every Sunday. She had daughters, and I became close to them. At Easter time, I went into town and bought ducklings for them to keep in the pond they had out back.

My mom never came to visit me until I had the baby, and my father came out just once. He brought me a little dog. I understood why they didn't want to visit me in all those months: I was bad and had done this really horrible thing that hurt everybody. I was so happy they didn't just cast me into the river or something. That's how bad I felt.

After four and a half months, I went to the hospital to have the baby, and it was a girl. I was told I wouldn't be able to spend any time with her. If you put a baby up for adoption, you can't see it. But after the birth I became hysterical and said I wanted to talk to Dr. Cranbrook. I told her, "I want to see my baby. I want to see my baby!"

So she said, "Let her see the baby. Bring the baby to her." When they brought her to me, I noticed that her fingernails were just like mine. She looked like her father, too; there was no mistaking that it was mine and Frankie's.

I spent seven days with her. Then came cousin Eli the lawyer, and out came my mother for the first time. They took the baby from me and got into the car, and I went back to the doctor's house in a separate car. The baby went away and I thought to myself, *I will never feel as unhappy in my entire life as I feel right now.* And it was the truth: I never ever felt the kind of hurt I felt that day.

Fast-forward a lifetime. I got married and had two sons and a whole life. Frankie and I stayed in touch. Never did I not feel love for my baby. Never did a day pass when I didn't think of her and wonder whether she was okay.

Fifty years later, I met her again.

I had gone into the National Adoption Service and filed papers, and I posted her stats—where she was born and the year and the hospital. I didn't even know her name.

She found me.

She'd had a wonderful life, wonderful parents, and they told her if she was ever curious about finding her birth mother, they would help her. It was this incredible high to know she was okay.

The first time I saw her, I wanted to look at her fingernails. I remembered her nail beds were just like mine. So when we met, the first thing I said was, "Let me see your hands." And they looked just like mine.

ABORTIONS

SHAINA When we first started working on the book, the hashtag #youknowme was trending. Do you remember that?

JULIA It was incredible to read their stories. I'm really glad that people are starting to talk about this.

I was fifteen; he was sixteen. **He said he didn't enjoy the feeling of using condoms and how they made his dick soft.** Obviously missing a proper sex-ed class, we both somehow believed that pre-cum wouldn't get me pregnant, and that the pull-out method would suffice. We were two poor kids with the pressures of sex all around us. I started skipping school to be with him because life felt easier within the walls of his older sister's tiny, two-bedroom apartment. Two months later, I realized that my period had not come and I was eating more. I finally got the courage and told my favorite cousin about the fear that lurked within my belly and then my aunt, who bought me a test.

I held the test in my hand for a while. Then I peed on the stick and a pink line appeared; faint, but bright enough to be true. My heart sank and my mind wandered to a million and one places: *How could I have let this happen? What could I do?*

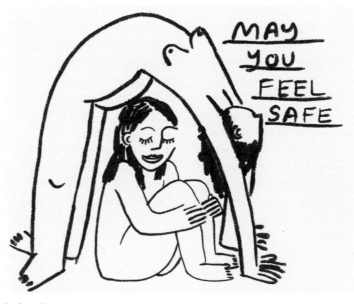

MAY YOU FEEL SAFE

Carissa Potter

Who would I become? What would he think? Could we be parents this young?

To soften the blow, my aunt told my mother. Thankfully she did, because the words could not find themselves within me. After the anger cooled down, my mom told me with a disappointed voice that I was scheduled for an

appointment a few weeks later.

I can still remember that day when I told him what happened, and how I wanted to crawl inside myself. He asked, "What are you going to do? I'm not sure what to tell you. It couldn't possibly be mine."

And I replied, "It's okay—my mom is handling it."

I was thirty-nine when I had an abortion. I've asked myself in the six years since why I didn't try not to get pregnant: *How I could I have been so reckless at an age when that excuse doesn't fly? And why had I fallen in love with someone so completely wrong for me?*

What I know: I'm a slow learner.

At the time, my daughters were four and six—tender things. **I was reeling from my divorce, ashamed for breaking apart my family. This new relationship was a chance to knit it back together.** Create an intact situation. Repair the damage.

L. was forty-three, never married, no kids. We were sexually compatible, mostly. We created our own island of intimacy and love, distant from reality. We talked about having a baby, even though we weren't yet living together. He wanted a child more than I did—someone to call his own in a world of what he perceived as leftovers.

I talked to my doctor about fertility on the cusp of forty. I took prenatal vitamins. We had unprotected sex. A lot of it.

Six months later, on a cold and rainy November day, a switch was flipped. I can't explain it any better than that, but I *knew*. And

for a woman who doesn't often know—a woman who lives in ambivalence more than clarity—I knew I could not have a child with this man.

That clarity came too late: a test the day before Thanksgiving confirmed the pregnancy.

Abortion, for me, was a lot about the loneliness leading up to it. The pain of telling your partner you've changed your mind. The ugly devastation that spreads over your entire existence.

Things I wondered in the weeks before as I took another test to confirm, told him in the kitchen surrounded by my favorite holiday foods, made the appointment, felt relief at having done so: *Am I fit to mother? What would my daughters think? Why am I so irresponsible? I should have known better.*

Things I've come to understand about myself since: I don't regret my decision. Of course I knew better, and still I made a mistake. I am now part of a cadre of women whose lives were forever changed by a choice. And I'm grateful it was mine to make.

In the clinic, he and I fought—because I took a call from my ex to arrange childcare, because I was doing this to him, because I

was taking something away. The woman shepherding me through asked if we needed more time; would I like to come back? I was adamant about having the abortion, even as he yelled, raged, left me to go pace in anger at a nearby bookstore, returned afterward, mute in the car, picking me up outside the clinic and dropping me off at home like he was my cabdriver, not my partner. Later, he brought a heating pad as an apology.

We stayed together another two years.

I don't regret the abortion. I don't regret ending the relationship, though I know I should have done so sooner. I am the proud mom of two amazing young women. My family, the three of us, is absolutely intact.

What do I regret? Not being able to speak my truth. Having to tamp it down in shame. Even today, when women are sharing their stories freely and with greater impunity, this—abortion at thirty-nine with no medical necessity, a pregnancy intended until it wasn't—feels verboten.

So let me say clearly and unapologetically: I had an abortion at thirty-nine. And it saved my life.

When I was seventeen years old, I had sex for the first time. This was pre-internet, and my mother never really talked to me about what it entailed, so I was pretty clueless. A boy liked me, I liked him, so I just thought this was the next logical step. He told me he would pull out, and I simply believed him. I don't even remember it feeling good. It was just something to do.

We'd had sex only a few times when I realized my period was late. My mother was the one who actually asked me, "Haven't noticed pads in the trash—anything you want to tell me?"

I didn't have any money. I asked my best friend if I could borrow money to buy a pregnancy test. I took it. It was positive. A few days later I asked another friend to lend me money, and I bought and took another test—still positive.

I called my boyfriend. I sobbed. He said next to nothing. He didn't want a baby. We agreed that me having an abortion was the only option. To say I was numb is an understatement. I was seventeen and living in Massachusetts, so it was illegal without parental consent. I called a clinic in Rhode Island and was told I could have the procedure there. I made an appointment.

I had no money. My boyfriend had no money. I was terrified of telling my parents. I called my brother. He gave me the money but told me I had to tell my parents.

I walked to the bus stop, as if I was going to school, and waited until my father drove away. Then I went back home and rang my own doorbell. My mother answered, saw my face, and said, "You're pregnant, aren't you?" She was disgusted by me. She thought I was trash. She told me I would never amount to anything now. My father came home and he cried.

I couldn't stay at home if I kept the baby—an embarrassment to my family. I had nowhere else to go. I told them my plan to go to Rhode Island with my boyfriend; an appointment had been made. It was to be the morning after my prom. I went to my prom thinking everything would be fine, and threw up on the side of the road.

In Rhode Island, at the clinic, I had to walk through protesters to get inside. They were yelling. I stood in line. I was crying. The woman next to me told me I would be okay. After I woke up, they gave me pretzels

and a ginger ale, and I threw up all over myself. I walked out to the waiting room, where my boyfriend had asked the girl next to him for her number.

My mother made me soup. I sobbed myself to sleep.

I got a registered letter in the mail. I don't remember if it was a few days or weeks later. It was from the clinic. My pathology results showed that I was still pregnant.

My mother stopped speaking to me. My father took me to the hospital. A nurse gave me an ultrasound. I didn't hear the sound, but I saw the flickering heartbeat. She left me alone in the room. My father and I met with the doctor. I can't recall anything about the conversation. I couldn't stop crying. Maybe I was worthless?

My father took me to the hospital the next day. My mother wouldn't take off from work. I was given a pill. I was told that it would hurt but would be okay. The operating room was cold. I was awake the whole time. The noises from the machine. The doctor telling me to stay calm, it would be over soon. A nurse on each shoulder because I was screaming and had to be held down.

Two weekends later, I went to my college orientation. My breasts started leaking and I had to squeeze them in the bathroom to relieve the pressure.

I am forty-four years old now, and the mother of two amazing children. I am truly happily married, and my husband listens each time I want to talk about this. I think about that baby almost every day—I'm not kidding, either. I am fiercely pro-choice and will forever fight for a woman to have whatever choice she wants.

But.

That baby would have been twenty-six years old today. I imagine a baby boy. Who would he have become? What would his life have been like? What if I'd gotten the support I so desperately needed and kept him? What did we miss out on by not being a family together? What if I had had him and given him to a loving family? The love that I feel for my children—surely I would have had the same for him?

I will forever think of that baby, and all the what-ifs. I love my children so fiercely—and I am a damn good mother—but I never gave him or me the chance together. I don't think I will ever forgive myself. I'm sorry...I'm sorry...please forgive me.

Right after I broke up with my boyfriend he said, "Let's have sex one more time." We fucked and I didn't realize but he came inside me. A couple months later, I I was feeling bad so I went to a health clinic. They had me pee in a cup. The nurse came back in the room and said, "You're pregnant." I contacted my ex and he happily told me, "You're gonna be a great mother and I'm gonna be a great dad." We went to an ob-gyn, and the nurse confirmed I was pregnant. Ten weeks. She told me I had a few months to have an abortion if I wanted.

I didn't think I had an option because of what he said. I told the nurse, "Of course I'll keep it. My boyfriend wants me to. What do I do next?" She looked at me and said, "Did you just say your boyfriend wants to keep it? I'm asking you. This is your choice. Do you want to have this baby?" I looked up at her and said no. I went back to the waiting room and told my boyfriend that I wanted an abortion. He got so mad and broke down.

But he still took me to the city to get it done. After it was over, he put me in a cab and told me he needed a drink. He said "I can't be with you. You killed my baby." I was in a lot of pain but I didn't regret it.

Today I am so thankful for that nurse. If it had been a different nurse, who didn't care to ask me like that, I would have had the baby. She was an angel. Also, one thing, I was a heavy smoker before this happened. But once I found out I was pregnant I stopped smoking. Even after it happened, I wanted it to mean something. So I haven't smoked a cigarette since that day. That was eighteen years ago.

Julia Rothman

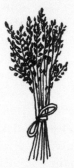

Revolutionary Outlaw Lovers

by **BIANCA I. LAUREANO, MA, CSES**

As a form of thanks, a client kissed my hand after the procedure. Another person was incarcerated, handcuffed to the bed, and didn't want to be touched, and I reminded them to breathe. Others want to hear a story, or what part of the termination process we are at and what comes next. Everyone is different, and everyone has their own needs and expectations.

Abortion doulas are people who sit with and support pregnant people experiencing an abortion. Yes, we support those who are making some of the hardest decisions of their lives. They too deserve compassion and empathy. They also deserve affirming, quality care.

Being an abortion doula means valuing body autonomy in some of the most radical ways. It requires me to remove myself and my own ideas and stereotypes of what a family means, what choice looks like in action, and how to navigate my own issues before showing up for someone else. In short, I must hold myself accountable. Accountability, body autonomy, and collaboration are what make being an abortion doula possible.

Often abortion doulas are trained in pain-management techniques—how the body responds to certain types of pain, ways to massage or touch people who are in a reclining position during a procedure. This training is often offered by pregnancy doulas, the kind of doulas that many people are more familiar with. These are full-spectrum doulas; they value the care that pregnant people need, regardless of their choice to parent. There are doulas for abortion, for adoption, and for birth.

Abortion doulas are often assigned to a particular location with clients. Some places are reproductive-health clinics; others may be hospitals. Of course, there are always abortion doulas in less formal settings, such as medication abortions or experiences of miscarriage.

The collaboration between medical provider and patient is where abortion doulas do their care work. In choosing this path of care work, I asked myself why I had not learned about abortion or care for those experiencing one in my professional development as a sexuality educator. We have separated the reality of abortion from the human-sexuality experience. I wanted to bridge that gap for my own knowledge and growth and because this is what my interpretation of mentorship looks like in action: expanding the US sexuality field to be more inclusive.

Imagine making one of the most difficult decisions in life—who would you want there with you? What if that decision challenged your relationship with your creator/universe/family/culture; who would you want by your side? Uncertainty about the answers to these questions is common. This is where abortion doulas find themselves: at the intersection of complicated care work.

Abortion doulas are not a new or modern care for supporting people through a pregnancy experience. Instead, abortion doulas are revolutionary outlaw lovers. *Revolutionary love* in the Chela Sandoval sense (that is, as a radical political ethic and methodology), and *outlaw* in the Dorothy Allison sense of *outlaw territory*: the common space women who are "outside the acceptable definition of what a woman is supposed to be" may occupy. Ergo revolutionary outlaw lovers, challenging the binary. This is where we find pleasure.

Realizing this new form of care and identity evolved for me. There were times when I wondered if the hour-long train ride followed by a forty-five-minute crosstown bus ride was "worth it" to (and for) me. I had already done doula training and a hospital/clinic volunteer training

to be here, and now I'm questioning this trip? Sure, I'd take the ride for my own care, but what drove me to do this for others? There was a lot of time to think, read, and watch people. I thought of the clients who were traveling alone and those who had support in the waiting area. How did each of us prepare for this day? I was making an intentional decision to do this care work twice a month, for free, and with total strangers! I realized this is what revolutionary love is made of: a love so radical and liberating that it is the love for life and self.

Preparing for a shift was always important. I would plan my schedule and know the night before that I had to get to bed by a certain hour to make sure I was not late if caught in rush-hour traffic. I planned for clothing that was easy to change out of (and into scrubs) once I arrived. Making sure I was not wearing any scents was important: I'm often right next to the client, near their head, and the last thing I wanted to cause was an allergic reaction during a vacuum aspiration! Breathing was a priority for clients, and I didn't want them to breathe in an artificial scent.

Scent was a part of the care work, but only if a client chose to be exposed to the lavender I brought with me. Selecting comfortable shoes was crucial, as I would stand near and with clients, sometimes sitting with them too. My body was a priority in this work as well. My relationship with (and care for) my body was a requirement to do this care work as an abortion doula. The outlaw emerged: caring for others required caring for myself, and that care was vital. Being an abortion doula brought me back into my body, and I was able to find new forms of pleasure.

Whenever I offered updates to a client's loved ones who had accompanied them, they too experienced relief. One family member hugged me and thanked me for sharing the news that their person was okay and recovering as expected. Another client's kin held my hand as they shared their fear in tear-filled Spanish. For them, abortion in their homeland often meant death: not only death for the pregnant person because abortion was illegal and frequently fatal, but also death for those who supported the abortion: doctors, doulas, partners. Knowing the complexities of immigration and migration from my own family's choices to leave their homeland, I know what is lost and what is gained. The revolutionary outlaw lover is a complicated and layered space where storytelling and listening lead.

Pleasure is a word for so many things! Choice is pleasure. Body autonomy in action with no barriers is pleasure. Having choice and body autonomy witnessed is a gift of pleasure. Using love as a political weapon that deeply guides our ethics and community collaboration is revolutionary. The love practice and experiencing pleasure simultaneously, collectively, is what body autonomy in action offers. This is also where abortion doulas find themselves: at the varied and brilliant space where pleasure expands.

Pleasure and love are powerful. Abortion doulas do not embody this power easily. I have to understand how power is at play during every part of the abortion and care process. I must ask myself hard questions that are often at the center of body autonomy and pleasure, yet rarely do we know to ask them.

Listed below are my core questions when creating boundaries for myself—boundaries not only of what is not possible, but boundaries to share what *is*. If I have the curiosity and self-awareness to ask these questions, hear the answers, and respond accordingly, then I am able to offer the care that is needed for each person during their abortion experience.

- Does this person want to be touched?
- How do I figure out how they want to be touched—just ask?
- How do I make this clear if we don't speak the same language?
- My hands are clammy—will they still hold and squeeze them?
- Do they feel like I'm hovering over them?
- What do I do with my body?

Being in your own body is a requirement for an abortion doula, given that we are using our bodies to be present and of support. It's a constant navigation into what is possible and what is happening. Preparation and care like this make me an amazing revolutionary outlaw lover! These hard questions about what is happening in my body and in theirs—about the power we are both using and holding—challenge a dehumanizing approach that is all too common in medical care for pregnant people. In listening to their responses, I am able to honor boundaries and body autonomy that may differ from my own. These are the new boundaries we create together, and it is a collaboration, a love for self. Revolutionary outlaw lovers.

A radical love for self-preservation is where a reproductive justice framework reminds us that we have the human right to have a child, not have a child, and parent the children we have. Reproductive justice is about pleasure in all the ways it may be experienced for each person, regardless of class, race, ethnicity, gender, immigration status, disability, or location.

Sometimes when making difficult decisions, we do not want an audience or witness. Other times we have no or limited choices. The agency within the constraints that abortion doulas affirm for pregnant people is so valuable. Experiencing abortion is a type of pleasure in practicing body autonomy and choice. Sometimes pleasure is more than we thought it could be. Sometimes pleasure is exactly what we choose and need. May we each experience the pleasure we desire on our own terms—and may we be given the gift of experiencing a revolutionary outlaw lover when needed!

Sources

Sandra Cisneros in Conversation with Dorothy Allison, 1996. Lannan Foundation. Available at: https://vimeo.com/9241859. Retrieved July 10, 2019.

Sandoval, Chela. *Methodology of the Oppressed.* University of Minnesota Press, 2000.

LIFE AFTER A SEXUAL ASSAULT

KAREN KORNEGAY

I t was 1996, and I was nineteen years old. I went to a club in Biloxi, Mississippi, called Mustang Sally. I was with my boyfriend—a guy I'd been dating for a while—and we were with friends. I didn't drink. I never drink. Everyone else started getting drunk, and as the night went on, my boyfriend started getting aggressive and handsy. He was angry at me because my outfit was attracting attention from other men. I had on a skirt and a black tank top. He'd been aggressive before, but it had never led to any sexual abuse. However, on this night, he started putting his hands up my skirt, saying, "I know this is how you like it, I'm just giving you what you want."

He grabbed my boobs, grabbed my ass, and I said, "Come on, just calm down. You've had a little too much. Why don't we get out of here? Go home?"

But he said, "No, I'm not done partying yet."

I told his friends he was getting handsy and rowdy. Then guys started approaching me because they knew it was pissing him off. My boyfriend kept getting madder at me. I said, "Let's go outside and take a breather."

We went out to the car—the club was on the beach, and we had parked all the way at the back. There was nobody else out there. By this time he was really angry at me. He told me that I shouldn't have dressed the way I did. And then he started pulling up my skirt.

I said, "This isn't cool. This isn't who you are."

He ripped my shirt, and I thought about how I couldn't go back into the club like that. Then he flipped me over and pushed me down on the car. I tried to calm him down. "You don't understand what you're doing. You're going to regret this in the morning. Please, please stop." I tried to flip back around so I could look him in his face and I kept repeating, "You need to stop. This isn't you."

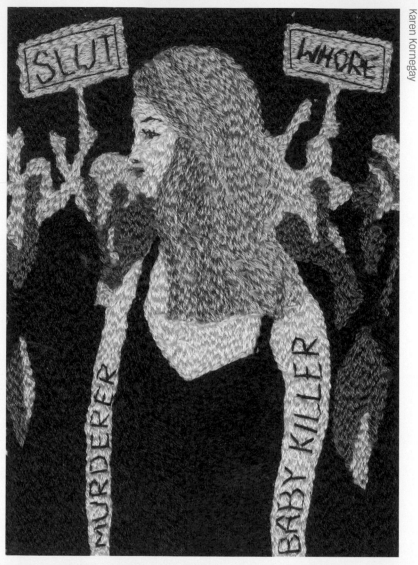

Karen Kornegay

He ripped off my underwear and then he raped me. I tried to move but I couldn't. He was really big and really strong. At first he entered me vaginally, but then somehow he stumbled and it came out, and as I tried to flip around he took me anally. His arm was underneath my face, so I couldn't even yell. At that point I just kind of went blank and numb and wanted it to be over with. I stopped saying no, but I do remember wondering, *Am I consenting if I don't keep trying to stop this?*

By that time my skirt was ripped off, my shirt was ripped off, my bra was gone. I think I kind of blacked out—passed out from shock. The next thing I remember, I woke up on the asphalt. His car was gone and there were cops in the parking lot. Someone asked, "Ma'am, are you okay?" I couldn't even think.

At the station, they did a rape kit and asked if I knew who did it, but I didn't tell them because I didn't want my boyfriend to get in trouble. I felt guilty. I felt like it was my fault, because I wore the clothes that triggered the attention that made my boyfriend mad in the first place. I thought I deserved for this to happen. I should have tried harder to stop him. Or I shouldn't have gone outside with him. Or knowing that he was getting handsy, I should've done something different.

Then I became pregnant. I knew there was no way I could have the child. I decided to go to an abortion clinic, and during the initial visit they gave me a little information session. They said, "It's a really easy procedure, very professionally done, and it's not painful to the baby." I didn't see any pictures or anything, but they did reassure me that it was quick and harmless, no big deal. The procedure would cost $300. Afterward, I had twenty-four hours to make my choice.

The day I went to have it done, there were tons of protesters outside. I had to pass through electric gates to get into the parking lot, but the protesters could still see me, and they yelled: "Baby killer! Murderer! Slut! Whore!" I think back now and there was nobody out there saying, "You're not a horrible person. Can I pray with you? You don't have to make this decision alone."

Inside the clinic, a nurse gave me the paperwork and said, "It's going to be quick. Don't worry about it." I don't remember every detail, but I remember the stirrups and the doctor inserting something. I remember feeling nauseous, like I was going to pass out. I kept asking the doctor questions. I wanted to know how much longer, and he refused to answer. He treated me like I was some meaningless person, like I wasn't even there. And when he was done, I started crying and shaking, and knew at that moment that I'd done something God would deem unforgivable.

The canister for the vacuum was on the left, so I turned my head to the right. I didn't want to see it. The doctor grabbed the canister and walked around to talk to the nurse, stopping inches from my face. At that point, I was broken. I felt like the worst person in the world. I was not deserving of anything, totally worthless, because I had chosen to take the life of a child. Actually it had been children—I found out I'd been carrying twins. Lying there, I thought, *I'm going to hell*.

There was nobody there to comfort me.

For a long time, I carried the names those protesters threw at me like an invisible chain around my neck. I thought there was no way God or anyone would ever forgive me for doing something so heinous and horrible. Since then, I've become a mom and now have four grown boys, but each time I had another child, I thought about how I had discarded those twins.

Then, four years ago, something changed. I was doing a Christian volunteer program inside an Alabama women's prison, and I met a couple of women on death row. One day we were doing a lesson on forgiveness and someone said, "God forgives everybody." It's hard to grasp that God could forgive even the unforgivable, but I felt these women prisoners needed to know that. And so I took their hands and said, "Look, I don't know what you've done, but God loves you no matter what and forgives you for what you've done." As it turns out, they were on death row for killing their children.

I remember praying about it, and I thought God was telling me, "If I can forgive even the worst of these people, what makes you think I can't forgive you?" Suddenly I felt a flood of emotion. I am not a crier, but I went to the chapel bathroom and broke down crying on the floor. That was the moment I let go of my guilt and shame—that chain around my neck fell away.

I am pro-life now. I struggle with identifying like this, and I also don't feel I have the right to tell anyone else what they should do. I just know the damage it caused me—my decision to have an abortion tortured me for a very, very long time. People might think I'm anti-women or anti-feminist because I'm pro-life, but that's not it. I just want other women to know there's another choice besides abortion. But I do struggle thinking about rape. I can speak to this because I've been through it and I know the after-effects are really, really difficult. And a baby is a baby. I would never make the same decision again.

Most of all, I hope my experience helps other women understand that they are not screwed up because they made this choice. They are not worthless. It does not define who they are.

Lastly, I have been able to forgive the guy who raped me. I know nothing about him now, and we haven't spoken a word since that night. He doesn't know I got pregnant, and he doesn't know I had the abortion. But if I saw him again, I would tell him that I forgive him. That's one of the hardest things—to forgive someone who has done something horrible—but it's part of the healing process.

And it's what set me free.

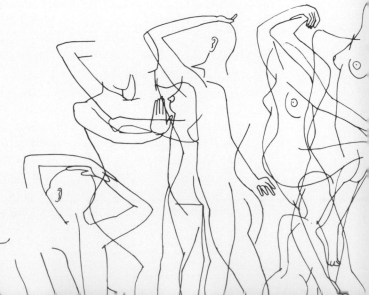

CONSENT & SEXUAL ASSAULT

SHAINA It was heartbreaking to hear from so many people about being sexually assaulted.

JULIA It was the topic that we got the most stories about. People need a place to share their experiences.

NOTE **If you or someone you know has been sexually assaulted, you can call the National Sexual Assault Hotline at 1-800-656-4673.**

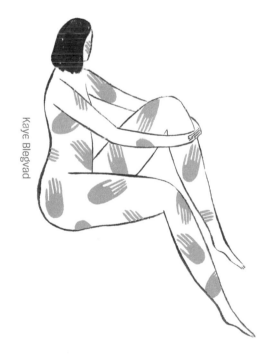

Kaye Blegvad

I think there is an element of feeling like, as a man, if someone wants to have sex with me, I'm supposed to want to have sex with them. **Sometimes I would have sex before I was ready or really wanted to.** I would think, *Somebody wants to have sex, so you should have sex.* Then I would feel bad afterward. So there has been something exciting about being able to say to sex partners these days, "Hey, I want to wait a while."

For the most part, this works out okay. But I have been in relationships where not being in the mood has conveyed to them something they're already feeling— because they feel bad about themselves. Which I don't want to do, either. So it feels fraught any way you go. The best situations I have found myself in are when I trust what the other person says, and I think they trust what I say. I've lied about wanting to have sex when I didn't. And I don't blame anyone else in that situation when that's happened. But it makes me so afraid that somebody could be feeling that way and I wouldn't know.

I was fourteen and had
a crush on a friend's older
brother. I invited him to my
house when I was home
alone. He brought beer and
friends. He spiked my
drink and raped me in
my mom's bed. That's how
I lost my virginity.

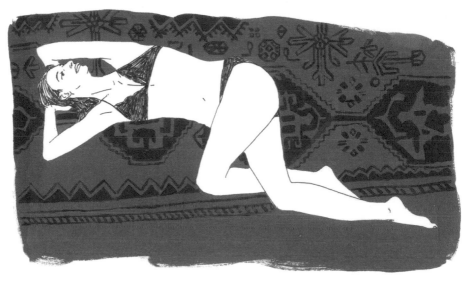

Julia Rothman

No was a word I said often to my high-school boyfriend.

I was sixteen years old and devoutly Christian. **In my mind, sex was a wonderfully sacred act that I was determined to save until my wedding night.** I could never imagine my life panning out any other way. In addition to my spiritual beliefs, I did not feel any desire to have sex at that age. These facts did not stop my boyfriend from pestering me to have sex with him every day.

One December afternoon I decided to take a shower at his house. His mother was gone and the two of us were alone. I felt comfortable in his home and safe with him. After all, he was my best friend. I loved him.

So when he entered the room while I was naked and drying off, I did not feel afraid. When he coaxed me to the bed and began to kiss me, I still did not feel afraid. When he suggested we have sex, I denied him as I always had. But this time he would not take *no* as an answer.

Memories of that event harbor in my mind to this day:

I remember frantically saying *no* at first, as though the power of that tiny word would repel him.

I remember him saying, "I'm already in—you might as well let me finish."

I remember falling silent and thinking, *This is it, I'm no longer a virgin; this is what it feels like.*

But most vividly I remember staring up at the popcorn ceiling until he was done. As he withdrew from me, he told me it was my fault: he could have made my first time romantic if I hadn't denied him so many times.

That was the first time he engaged in nonconsensual sex with me. Sometimes I would cry, sometimes I would fake orgasms to please him, and other times I was silent—but each time I would tell him *no*.

This event marked the beginning of my chronic depression and created an abyss between me and God that I have since learned to overcome. Long after that boyfriend stole what was precious to me and moved on to another love interest, swarms of questions ate at my soul:

Was it rape? It was not violent, as TV and sex education told me it would be.

Why did I just lie there? I should have screamed and pushed him off.

Why did I keep letting him have sex with me? I must have wanted it.

The truth is, I was young and confused. It took me many years to understand that what he had done to me was wrong. Our relationship status was not a consensual contract that dictated his right to have sex with me. It was never my fault.

I was nineteen and stoned and eating at an IHOP on Christmas Eve with my friend, and I told him, "Once at summer camp, my camp counselor made me masturbate in front of everyone in the cabin."

And he said, "Don't tell anyone that story."

When you're a kid, you just take experiences as they come. **You walk around the world and the adults are in charge.** I was twelve, and the topic of conversation among the boys in that cabin was, "Do you have sperm when you masturbate?" And I said I did. The counselor, who was probably seventeen or eighteen, overheard the conversation and said, "Prove it right here, right now."

Only when I revisited that story in IHOP did I realize how bad it was. I feel responsible and worried now, since he was a camp counselor and maybe he's still around hurting more kids. But at the time I was too afraid to do anything. I eventually told a detective who was a friend of the family and they checked the camp, but there hadn't been any other complaints.

I still know someone who was in that cabin with me. I could ask him tomorrow if he remembers that counselor's name, and I could do something, I guess. I just don't have the courage. I should. I will. If it's in my power to stop it, I should.

I worked on a farm in my hometown during summers off from college. **I loved how strong my body became and the praise I got for working my ass off.** But the middle-aged men around me saw it differently. The foreman was mean and built like a bull. He used to call me *dirty girl* as a joke, then *dirty bitch* when he decided to take it further.

"Too far," I told him.

He backed off for a while, until one afternoon he caught me in the pack shed as I was washing my hands at the end of a long hot day. His habit was to down a six-pack before he drove home for the night. He bent me over the sink and breathed in my ear. "How do you like that, dirty girl?"

My mind raced as I struggled to stand up—I was helpless against his strength. His broad arm pushing across my back, his stupid laugh.

"Stop! Get the fuck off me!"

Lucky for me, the farmer's wife walked by and yelled for him to quit it. Like calling off an attacking dog. He let go and walked away. I was nineteen then; he was fifty-five. The next morning, after getting a talking-to from the boss, he gave me a sheepish apology.

I worked there, with him, for another two summers. I even hugged him goodbye on my last day on the farm. I thought it was all part of the price you pay to do the work you love. Now I know better.

I was in my late twenties. I went into a job interview with a sculptor whose work I liked. He was really well-known. He had done all this research on me and knew I could make molds. I'm a straight guy and knew he was gay, but I didn't think anything of it. He gave me some wine after he showed me his studio. And then I realized he had roofied me.

I started feeling really queasy. He was just watching me and waiting until I passed out. I knew what was happening. I saw him kind of coming for me, and I just hit him. He was wrestling me and pulled me to the ground. I thought, *I have one chance,* so I hit him in the gut, ran out, and got in my truck.

I don't remember getting home, but I passed out at home and slept for a whole day. The fucked-up part was he had my résumé with my address. I guess a bracelet of mine had fallen off during our fight, so he mailed it back to me. Then he kept emailing me, inviting me to parties. I didn't report him, because what proof did I have besides my word against his?

A year ago, he committed suicide. I thought about telling my story then, but what justice would that serve?

On my mom's side I am one of many girl cousins, except for the oldest who is a boy. **He is twelve years older than me, and my whole childhood I idolized him and loved him more than anyone.** My immediate family and I lived across the country, and we would visit my extended family a few times a year and for long periods in the summers.

Whenever I was in town, he would go out of his way to spend time with me, taking me places and showering me with attention. He would dote on me, whisper in my ear that I was his favorite, and tell me how much he loved me. We would cuddle and were always very physical. He was charismatic and charming, but also wild; he lived a crazy life, with lots of girlfriends and drugs.

He would break my heart again and again when he wouldn't show up at family functions when he said he would, and I would wait and wait. One summer when I was sixteen, it became sexual. He was testing the waters, and I responded. At eighteen I had my first serious boyfriend and sex for the first time, but not long after that I had sex with my cousin. I'm glad he knew better than to be my first, at least. We carried on a secret love affair for many years.

He has always said I'm the love of his life. He wanted to marry me and make our relationship known, and I almost did it. My mom's family is an immigrant family—a prominent family

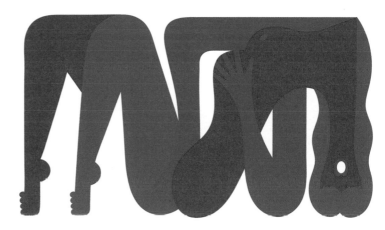

Olimpia Zagnoli

bloodline back home—and even my parents' generation has first cousins who are married. The first time my twelve-year-old cousin held me as a baby, he told my mom he loved me more than anything, and my mom told him, "Well, grow up and get a good job, and maybe you can marry her!"

My grandmother, the matriarch of the family who we were all very close to, knew about our relationship and said if it was up to her and it was the old days, she would make it happen.

In the end, I couldn't go through with it and had to end it. My father was from a different culture, and doing so would have alienated him and that side of the family. I was worried what people in general would think. It had always had a fantastical quality to it—always a secret, always sneaking away to places and hotel rooms. A lot of drugs.

And deep down I felt something was wrong with how young I was through it all.

I see my whole life—every relationship, every choice to this day—through the lens of my relationship with him. Everything is affected by it. I feel like it, and he, had a big part in shaping who I am. I still hold his love as the love that all others compare to.

It's problematic for me. I feel he was much older than me and should have known better. That I never had a choice. And sometimes I wonder when exactly it became sexual for him. Although I would never go back to that kind of relationship with him, I still love him as family; we are still very close, and he is still one of the most important people in my life. Is it a tragic love story or a story of incest and abuse? I'm still not sure.

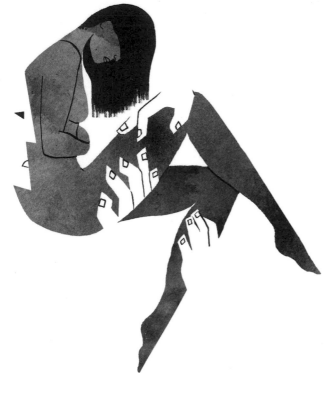

Hanna Barczyk

When I was sixteen I had my first boyfriend. I was obsessed with him. I thought he was the love of my life, as sixteen-year-olds do. **We went to boarding school, and over one of the breaks I went to visit him and his family.**

I was sleeping in their family guest room, and I woke up in the middle of the night and he was having sex with my body. I wasn't conscious, so I hadn't consented. But rather than let him know I was awake, I just pretended to stay asleep. The next day I woke up, and it was the day I was going home, and I just didn't think about it.

In fact I never thought about it until I mentioned it in therapy one time, and then it all came out. I hadn't thought about it as *rape* for so long—because we were sixteen, and because we were in a relationship. But then I realized it was.

Now I feel—not over it, but I've made peace with it. And I tell people the story because I feel like staying silent means that I'm ashamed of it in some way. I hope it helps other people to hear about it. I told the story to a room of 200 people—for this sexual-awareness event at business school—and all of these other people got up and told their stories. It's really eye-opening how many people have had this happen to them.

These days with consent, I almost feel like you gotta record something. I text a girl sometimes and want her to say over text, "Yes— I want to have sex with you." I'm worried about that one crazy chick who lies and says, "I didn't tell him that—he raped me." I've heard it too much. **If the cops ask, then I have a text message to prove it.**

My ex-boyfriend recorded us having sex without my permission. We were a little wasted, and I didn't see he had a phone out and was recording us.

A couple of days later I saw it on his phone, and I was really insulted. It broke us up.

An open letter to all those who suffered sexual abuse as children:

Dear Survivors,

I was eight years old when my virginity was taken from me.

The "minor" occurrences of sexual abuse started as early as I can remember. I remember the 1970s decor like it was only yesterday. I remember being kissed in the kitchen, feeling his teeth sticking into my lips and face and him forcing his tongue into my mouth. It was because he loved me, he said. Most of the touching happened on his knee in the living room, in front of a clapped-out gas fire and a sunburst clock in faux brushed metal on the wall. It was our little secret, he said.

I was unceremoniously thrown off him as soon as we heard the familiar creak of the back door, as my grandma walked in from shopping at the market. I remember the feeling of grazing my knee on the cheap, patterned carpet and thinking about how I threw my dolls on the floor. I remember my grandma sliding open the inner door and giving me a look that I didn't understand. I was five years old. She knew and did nothing.

The worst of his offenses happened in their downstairs toilet, where he would ask me to do things to his half-naked body. When I was eight, he started doing more invasive things to me. Wood panels on walls make me shudder for too many reasons.

After the sex stopped and I became more aware that what he'd done to me was wrong, he started to make threats: I would be responsible for the family falling apart if I said anything to anyone. All of it would be my fault. I believed him for too long.

I'm sharing my story for all the children who have had their virginity and innocence taken from them too soon, whether they are still kids now or long grown up. The abuse that I suffered for almost my entire childhood played a part in shaping the person I am today. But it will never define me completely.

If you're surviving anything similar to this, hopefully you'll understand and come to know that you are so much more than your horrible experiences and memories; they are a part of you, but they are not the whole of you.

My parents found out what happened to me when I was twenty-one. Thankfully, it was then that my long road to recovery began. My mum cut ties with my grandparents, and in the process saved my life. My step-granddad died when I was twenty-six. I started therapy at thirty-five. I am now thirty-seven.

My plea for anyone out there in a similar situation is to not suffer in silence. If this is happening to you, tell someone. *Now.* And if they do nothing about it, tell someone else. I know that talking about it can be the hardest thing to do, but it might just be the moment that you no longer have to endure any more pain.

I see you and I'm with you, even if I don't know who you are or where you are in the world. Sadly, there are hundreds of thousands more just like us. But that also means that there are many more people on this planet who know how you feel—and they have survived. No matter how hard it gets (and recovery is a very difficult path to tread), there is life on the other side of your abuse.

I promise.

Yours sincerely,

B

When I was thirty-three, my brother ruined my outwardly perfect family's Waspy Episcopalian Thanksgiving by declaring to me (in front of my sister and his wife) that he'd been molested as a child (by another older boy) and that he in turn had molested me.

I had no memory of this.

My brother is a *cowboy*—like, literally a rancher. The epitome of desirable manhood. **He's tall, he's handsome, he's a fucking Marlboro man without the cigarettes.** I, manifestly, am not. I am bookish, introverted, and obviously gay to anyone with half an attention span, despite desperate youthful attempts to hide this reality from myself and everyone around me. And I grew up tortured by the specter of his perfect manliness that I could never quite fake.

Because of this, I grew up highly conflicted about my sexuality. I always knew I was gay, but I also "knew" that *should not* be true. (Growing up gay in a Christian family in the South will do that to you.) I was never able to connect with the men that I desired. I was hesitant to approach men I was attracted to because I wasn't sure what I wanted, and I didn't want any concrete proof that I wasn't straight, *just in case.*

What I didn't know was that my childhood experience at the hands of my perfect, Paul Newmanesque masc brother had given me PTSD about any sort of physical intimacy. When men would express interest, I would physically and emotionally freeze, then sort of black out; later I would come to, wondering why things hadn't gone more smoothly. I didn't come out until I was twenty-six, and I wasn't with another man in any meaningful way until I was thirty.

The worst moment of my entire life was the conversation when I was informed that I'd been

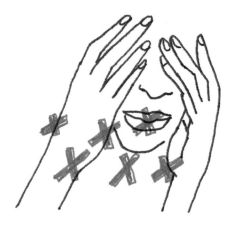

molested as a child. I didn't know and hadn't remembered, and the feeling that a key piece of my life experience had been hidden from me was devastating. So many embarrassing experiences suddenly made sense! It also meant I had to replay every part of my life for thirty years and reevaluate all I'd lost, all I'd missed out on, and all that I'd been unable to enjoy because I wasn't in charge of my own story.

On balance, however, it was the most freeing, empowering thing I've ever experienced. After two years and extensive (and expensive) therapy, I'm landing on my own feet. I feel confident in my body, and I am learning confidence in relationships with people I'm attracted to. The work has been hard, but I feel empowered, and deeply grounded in my emotions. My relationships are rich and full and broad in a way I never knew was possible.

I'm working hard to own myself; to release my (misplaced) shame and frustration; and to connect with people whom I love and trust. Every day brings a small victory among setbacks. But the shame is going (if not gone), and forgiveness is possible.

The best part? I have patience and empathy for everyone "weird" around me, because I know what it's like not to feel in control of your own story. It's a richness born of a robbery.

I was at college; it was the 1960s. It was my freshman year. I had experience making out with boys, but I'd never seen them naked. I made some friends my first semester. A lot of them were going to fraternity parties.

One of my friends in my suite had a boyfriend, and they invited me to a party with this guy. We went to the party and had a good time. We were making out at the party. He wanted to see me again, so he asked me out on a date. I said okay. I think he was wealthy; he had his own car at school.

He picked me up, and I don't remember what we did. We probably went out for dinner somewhere. We were in the car on the way back, and he drove into a dark parking lot.

I said, "Where are you going?"

He said, "I thought we could just stop here for a while and fool around."

He stopped the car, and when I looked over at him his pants were open and his penis was fully erect. I got really scared. I was shocked.

I said, "Whoa, put that away. Let me out of here."

And he said, "No, shhh, don't get upset. Just touch it."

And I said, "No—let me out. Let me out!" I tried to open the door.

He said, "Where you gonna go?"

There was nothing around. I tried to open the door again and he said, "Okay, okay," and zipped up his pants.

And I said, "Take me back."

I couldn't look at him the rest of the way home. And I never went out with him again.

It was my first or second week of freshman year of college. **My friend's brother was a senior and in a fraternity, and he invited us to a party. I was really excited to go.** I went with a few of my friends. We started drinking. I didn't drink in high school, so I didn't realize how drunk I was getting. Everything became a bit hazy. Some guy made an announcement: "Who wants to kiss this lovely girl?" I think about four or five different guys came over and kissed me.

Then the same brother of my friend who invited us—and who I thought was supposed to protect us—took me upstairs. There was a big mattress overlooking a window. He laid me down on the mattress and started making out with me and feeling me up. Eventually he took off all my clothes. I remember not wanting him to. I couldn't really respond because I was pretty drunk. I know I said "No, I don't want to do this" at some point, but he kept pushing me.

Other people were walking by. I was so embarrassed to be naked and have them all see me, but I felt like I couldn't get up. Other guys stopped by the room and touched and kissed me. Then my friend's brother forced me to have oral sex with him. He put his dick in my mouth and thrust it in and out. He kept saying, "Keep it open. Open it up." He also gave me oral sex.

When he started to put on a condom, I remember saying, "Please no, please no," and then I started crying. That's when he stopped. He looked at me and said, "Get your clothes on. I'm going to take you home." And then he actually did walk me back to my dorm.

I've never told anyone this story, except for my sister.

FORENSIC SEXOLOGIST

ERIC GARRISON

When I was a child, Dr. Ruth Westheimer had a radio show. And because she used these words that are really quite benign—like *penis*—her show was allowed to air late at night. So I would listen to her show in my childhood home in Richmond, Virginia. It was something like Mondays from midnight until 2 a.m. And I saved up my money from mowing lawns or from birthdays, and I bought a little digital clock radio, and I'd slide it under my pillow at night because I wanted to hear what advice she gave people on how to have better sex.

I just fell in love with her—her grandmother-type voice, her acceptance of differences. She wasn't overly conservative, and she made people laugh and think and feel okay about themselves; that was something else that I found positive about her. That was what I wanted to do.

That was when I was really young—before high school. Then in college I became a peer educator and learned more about how to educate people about sex. And eventually I got a degree in sex research in London.

Sex just fascinates me! It does so many wonderful things for the human body. And sex can function in so many ways—it can be an expression of love, friendship, lust. It can boost the immune system. It creates intimacy, it can be bonding. In some couples, there's the chance of procreation. It provides so many different things for so many different people!

I wear many different hats. I am an author, a speaker, a sex counselor. I have a private practice where I counsel clients on various issues of human sexuality and sexual growth and development, for their relationships or as individuals. A lot of my time is spent doing trauma-informed work with survivors. And I am a forensic sexologist, which means I appear in court for various sex-related cases. I help determine whether it was a sexual assault or a stalking or an issue of intimate partner violence. A lawyer will call me to look at documents and hear testimony to help determine what happened sexually. Sometimes it involves court appearances, sometimes it's just helping a lawyer with their case.

I've been doing forensic sexology about twenty years now. A lot of times, a perpetrator will claim that it was consensual strangulation. Then I explain to the court about BDSM and how what they are describing is not consensual. So sometimes I'm providing definitions, and that helps the judge further understand the case.

Something that people don't readily recognize is that BDSM has some of the most thorough forms of consent. If you think of a BDSM relationship—with a dominant and a submissive or a dominant and a slave, or a top and a bottom, whatever terminology you want to use—you think that the top is the one with the power, but really it's the bottom. The bottoms are the ones who say, *I consent to this. I give you the power to do this.* So even when they give up power, they are the ones who are saying, *I have this power to give up.*

In many BDSM relationships there are safe words, or there's what we call a *stoplight system.* There's a green-light word, which means *Keep going.* They have a yellow-light word (or a hand signal), which means *Slow down, not so deep, not so hard.* And they have a red-light word, which means *Stop* or *I need to catch my breath or recover for a while.* And then there's a black-out word—like, *This isn't doing anything for me, We need to stop, I need to go home,* or *You need to go home.*

Many people don't understand that BDSM is one of the more consensually based relationships out there. So sometimes a perpetrator of a sex crime will say, *This is consensual, this is what we do.* And I'll have to say, *I'm sorry, but this doesn't fit into the definition of consent,* or *Yes it does.* Sometimes it's just that someone says, *This was choking.* And I'll be pulled in to say, *This is extremely violent; this is nonconsensual strangulation, not choking.*

Typically, strangulation is a sign of potentially lethal behavior—a sign of a very violent person. So strangulation is a signifier that things could become more violent later.

Often when a sex crime comes up in the media, I get interviewed about it. Recently I was interviewed by a magazine about sexual grooming; after that interview, people called me from all over the world simply because they wanted to share their personal stories of sexual grooming. *Sexual grooming* is when a person will build trust in a potential victim so that they will consent to something that they don't really consent to. The perpetrator will break this person down, and break down their support systems, over a long period of time. Often the victim didn't even realize they were being groomed.

Since 1987 I've been speaking to college students about sex and sexuality. I give them index cards, then have them write a myth about human sexuality on one side and a question they've always wanted to ask on the other. The goal is to inspire them to ask a question about sexuality.

But to get them thinking and writing, I have them write out a myth about some aspect of human sexuality. I've been fascinated by the fact that in twenty-five years I've gotten the same question over and over from 250,000 college students: *Am I normal?* They ask it in different ways, but they all want that sexual affirmation. I don't like the word *normal,* so I always talk about how things are natural, not normal. *That's natural,* is what I say. *It's natural to have a variety of sexual desires.* And when I say that, people relax.

As a sex counselor, I address various topics in my private practice—erectile concerns, ejaculatory concerns, lack of desire. I see couples for discordant desire a great deal—where someone wants to have more sex, or where both partners want to have the same amount, but at different times or in different ways. So how do we deal with that? I usually recommend that we stop thinking about the goal of sex as orgasm. So many people think *sex* means *orgasm.* But if we make it about pleasure, it makes it easier for them to optimize the experience. I invite and inspire couples to find pleasure in providing pleasure. For example, I may hate to rub my partner's feet, but I love it when my partner is happy. So if I rub my partner's feet and they are happy, and then they start touching themselves—that's a form of sex. It's not just about sex organs merging together.

Sex is complex. And it really benefits people to widen their definition of what sex is.

I hear many questions from breast-cancer survivors and their partners. Sometimes it's a survivor who's had a mastectomy or a double mastectomy, and they come to me and say, "I miss my tits." I had a woman say to me, "I loved my tits. I miss them. I want to have a funeral service just for my tits." Then there are the partners who see the breast-cancer survivor as fragile—they've been taking care of that person for months—years, sometimes—and it's often hard for the partner to switch their caregiver brain off. The survivor is saying, "Please fuck me!" And the caregiver is thinking, "I don't want to hurt you!" So I talk to those people and tell them it's okay to acknowledge the survivor's consent to fuck them!

I also field questions from people who are interested in expressing their sexuality in a new manner—people who are coming out as interested in a kink or a fetish. And for those people, here's my advice: *lean in.* Instead of diving into the deep end of BDSM, just lean in; dip a toe in. Instead of building that dungeon in your basement, start off reading some BDSM erotica. I find it's easier to wade in than to take the plunge. And I tell them to be present, to honor where you are on that journey. I say, *Don't let fear be your guide; find something positive to lead you.*

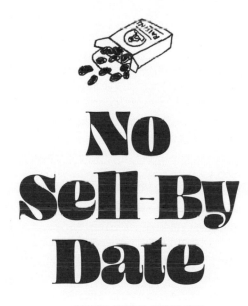

No Sell-By Date

by **GRETTA KEENE, LCSW, CST**

It happened on a long drive across the desert when I was four years old. I had to go to the bathroom, the next gas station was miles away, and I refused to go by the side of the road. My mother told me to pull my panties up tight in my crotch to hold in the pee.

Wowee!

Thus began a nightly exploration of the electrically charged button between my legs. As the years passed, I added sexual scenarios to my mastery of those exciting and soothing sensations. My best friend's discovery of her mother's hidden stash of *True Confessions* and her father's col-

lection of *Playboy* stored under the bed added to the repertoire. My friend and I "fooled around," excited by the forbidden secrets. Shame was the threat, but it sure felt good. Over sixty years later, it still feels good.

My mother—long divorced, wheelchair-bound, and on oxygen—would send me to the Body Shop to buy her mango butter, the coconut-rich cream she found most suitable for masturbation (and now preferred to her old standby, Vaseline). Accompanying her on many doctor's visits, I would also be in charge of explaining her adamant decision to avoid taking an SSRI for her depression because it cut down on her ability to give herself an orgasm. She was considered an old woman. The doctors' response to her stubborn stance ranged from mild amusement to incredulity and disgust. She refused to feel shame. Some things, both pleasure and comfort, like coffee and cookies, she refused to give up. I get it. Simple pleasures and comforts make the hard stuff worth doing.

Sexual liveliness has no automatic sell-by date. Our concepts of pleasure and comfort evolve and expand from childhood's breast-sucking, ice cream–licking, hug-seeking, pantie-pulling desires to satisfying and loving sexual connections with other pleasure- and comfort-seeking adults. But life can lead in another direction. My husband and I, both psychotherapists, see couples as a couple. We know that sexual aliveness can wither from shame and confusion or lack of opportunity, attention, skill, and trust. Wounding experiences and distorting beliefs can lead to toxic behaviors that poison rather than nourish, disconnecting the person from others and their own vitality. Resigned acceptance of diminished aliveness evolves into entrenched habits of denial. Life can seem a determined march across a landscape of expectations and responsibilities. We lose touch with curiosity and delight. The desire for pleasure and physical connection gets shoved into a dark closet. But like plants seeking the sun, we grow toward those surprising cracks where the light gets in.

My prim and proper, Southern lady, ninety-four-year-old paternal grandmother got nabbed in the nursing home for "inappropriate behavior" when her hand got stuck down the pants of her "beau." They were an item on the floor for mild dementia, and she told me with adorable coyness when I brushed her hair and helped her dress that she liked to look nice for her "admirer." Smitten, he would maneuver to sit next to her in the common room, tell her she was beautiful, and help her with her walker. At mealtimes, she would give him her olives. They were found more than once in each other's rooms, awkwardly attempting to add skin contact to their passionate embraces. I was called in by the staff and told that they would be kept separate via vigilant chaperoning because their behavior was both unseemly and against the rules. I argued on their behalf to no avail. Isolated from that spark of aliveness, my grandmother and her beau sank further into a despondent fog of dementia. One day she cried, "Why am I still here?" There were no more reasons for her to be alive.

When I was approaching the dreaded "change," I wrote a paper entitled "Embracing the Crone Through the Fire of Menopause." My friends were aghast and declared they were going to do everything possible to forestall the inevitable witchy identity. "But postmenopausal can be incredibly sexy!" I argued. "In Celtic tribes, the women past childbearing age were in charge of sexually initiating the young men. The seasoned women were considered experts, and their tutelage cut down on young bucks impregnating young virgins not ready to be mothers." My friends were not convinced.

There are many ways to dance the energetic whirl we call *life* that lead to joy and satisfaction. Our dance of aliveness manifests itself through what we do and how we connect to other forms of aliveness. Sexual aliveness is not dependent on attractiveness to another human, yet that quality is recognizable to others. It can be culturally confusing to feel attracted to the twinkle in the eye of the exuberant and emotionally warm older man or woman. Age is not a factor. Our spirit responds to those whose vitality shines through the outer cloak of body. The trick is to stay fully alive while you *are* alive; the years pass fast.

I'm lucky. I know that. Only a decade younger than when my mother died, I have an abundance of what makes my life worth living. I like, love, respect, and desire my husband. He tells me (often) that he feels the same way toward me. We work together and have fun together. Even though our lives are busy and our bodies have been around for nearly seven decades, we enjoy the happy dance of a satisfying and passionate sex life.

A harmonious and emotionally nourishing relationship requires two people committed to addressing old traumas, ingrained habits, and misguided and overactive defenses that shut down vulnerability and awareness. What we say and what we do either reinforce the old useless and destructive behaviors or enliven our emotional and energetic ties. A relationship generously salted with affection, appreciation, and regular acts of courtship creates an environment conducive to the delicious sharing of exciting and satisfying sexual pleasures. Kitchen hugs, garden kisses, hands held, dishes washed—all of these count.

"The raisin experience" is often part of an introduction to mindfulness and holds the key to great sex—no matter the age. Here's the deal: The mindfulness teacher tells everyone to close their eyes and hold out their tongue, on which an unknown object will be placed. (It is a raisin.) They are instructed to do nothing more at first than to consider the object on their tongue. Then, with intense focus, slowly roll the object with the tongue, taking in all its qualities, letting go of all judgment. Next, gently squeeze the object between the teeth and focus on the flavorful juice emitted. With the tongue, push the object to the roof of the palate and observe both texture and taste. Explore the object slowly and mindfully, again suspending judgment. When random thoughts drift in, return focus to the physical sensations of the raisin—each chew carefully noted, the interaction between object and mouth observed. Eventually only the taste is left. Hold that awareness until no flavor is discerned.

This process can take quite a long time. There is no rush. The point is to experience each moment with curiosity and appreciation, not critical analysis. Even if you think you don't like raisins (I didn't), let go of previous associations. Be vulnerable, open to surprise.

When treating a body part like a raisin, you might want to be careful what you chomp. But the idea is the same: Relinquish judgment and previous associations as much as possible. Focus intensely on the physical aspect of the touching body parts as you adventure. Rediscover that initial sensation of "Wowee!" and don't be afraid to say "Ouch!" A playful, inquisitive child-mind helps to dispel the cultural filters embedded with images of what we should look like and feel like, as well as past sexual experiences that can crowd out and distort the present moment.

Be vulnerable, open to surprise. Dry vulvas and soft penises can be coaxed into having a lot of fun. Initial pain and embarrassing discomfort can lead to unexpected, mind-blowing pleasure if greeted with patience and loving, trusting affection. Happy, mindful sex works well when there is a pleasure-giver and pleasure-getter in the first act, roles are reversed in the second act, and in the third act it's "Let's all come together! Right now!" Make dates to be spontaneous. Yes. Use it or lose it, but know that *lost* does not mean *gone forever.*

Don't wait until after dinner.

Be daring.

Engage all the senses. Mix candles and music, showers and baths, scents and silks (or whatever turns you on) with gusto and a sense of humor. If you can't find mango butter, coconut oil works. Welcome the opportunity to explore inner and outer landscapes.

A raisin is never too wrinkly, and neither are our bodies. Alone or with someone else, enjoy!

AGING

SHAINA I feel like the word *aging* has so many negative connotations, but some of the stories we got were really positive.

JULIA I'm still scared of getting old.

SHAINA You're scared of everything.

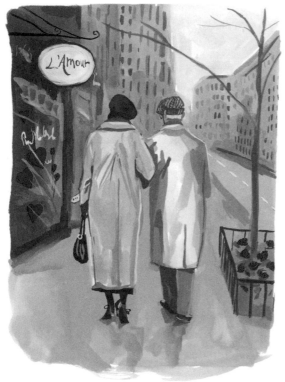

Jenny Krolk

I am seventy-three years old. After my divorce I had a partner for twenty years I did not marry or live with, but to whom I was very committed. He died many years ago. I then had several relationships but have been without a serious commitment. I no longer think much about having a partner or even dating.

This year three men have approached me to have an affair. Each is married. Two have known me for years, and I have always been aware of their interest in me.

I do not have an inclination to engage with a married man, but it sure makes me feel good to have been approached. Sometimes at night when I think about being older and the loss of my physicality, I remember that some men find me attractive and I giggle with delight.

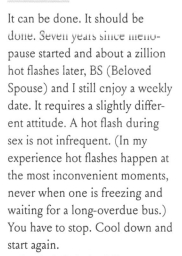

I've never had an orgasm!

I've never had mango!

I'm going through menopause right now. **I sweat a hell of a lot and have hot flashes, but sex is better!** It's better because first of all, I don't have a period—I can do it anytime, anywhere. And it's easier to reach that climax.

I loved going into menopause because it put the spontaneity back in my life. Before then, my husband and I had a hard time with birth control—figuring out the right one for us. And we had six pregnancies, which resulted in four kids. So once I went through menopause, we didn't have to worry about that anymore—and that felt great.

People said, "You'll get fat during menopause." But I was already fat! In fact, I got thinner. And we didn't lose our spark—feeling freer made things more fun for us. We didn't have to worry so much. The hot flashes weren't bad either—I've always been cold! My whole life I was cold.

I was forced into menopause because in my early fifties I needed to have a hysterectomy, so it happened very, very fast. It happened overnight for me.

It can be done. It should be done. Seven years since menopause started and about a zillion hot flashes later, BS (Beloved Spouse) and I still enjoy a weekly date. It requires a slightly different attitude. A hot flash during sex is not infrequent. (In my experience hot flashes happen at the most inconvenient moments, never when one is freezing and waiting for a long-overdue bus.) You have to stop. Cool down and start again.

Sex is definitely different. **It requires more of everything: time, stimulation, lubrication—especially the latter.** And the eventual payoff is much less intense. It becomes more about paying attention, but in a long-term relationship that's a good thing. It's still a good thing.

I got Viagra off this website. A friend referred me to it so I got it, and it really didn't do nothing for me. Maybe it was fake, I don't know. Then as I got older, I found out I could just go to my doctor and tell him I have erectile dysfunction (even though I don't). They can't test you for that! They write you a prescription right then and there.

You pop one in, and it's pretty good. Your penis stays hard for a long period of time. And even when you come, it just stays hard. It's almost automatic. It's almost instant. When you think about having sex, it gets hard. Normally you have to work up to it or get in the mood, but when you take Viagra you just think about sex and *bam*, it's there. It's there when you need it.

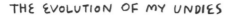

THE EVOLUTION OF MY UNDIES

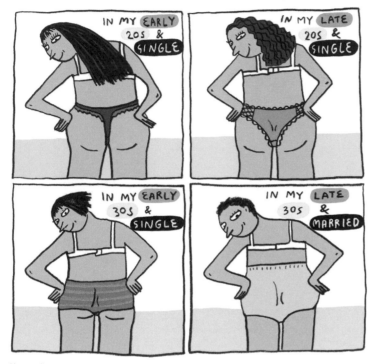

Hyesu Lee

I was with a female I wasn't physically attracted to, and I was unable to perform. I was confused; that had never happened to me before.

It's easy to say I wasn't attracted to her, but maybe it was me? I'm not looking forward to experiencing that again. I hear it's common, but I don't want it to be common.

Menopause sucks. I was lucky because after menopause I still got wet and still have a healthy sex drive, but it killed my body: I got scaly skin. I lost some vibrancy. I lost a youthfulness. It started at fifty, and then that was it. I got bad hot flashes. **You don't picture yourself old or feel old.** But you hit this wall.

COVID-19

JULIA We finished the book and handed it in and then...

SHAINA Coronavirus!

JULIA So we gathered some stories from people in quarantine and it turns out...

SHAINA ...there's lots of sexting during a pandemic!

My girlfriend and I met about a year before corona hit, but we didn't start dating until about a month before it really took off. **We had two dates right before the lockdown, and we were both excited to be starting something new. We hadn't had sex yet.** About two weeks into the pandemic, we joked about quarantining together, but we didn't. And once the shelter-in-place order became official, we quarantined apart for six weeks. We texted and FaceTimed a lot, told jokes, sent videos back and forth. It was kinda fun and felt like a throwback to courting, but it wasn't exactly fulfilling. Then, on April 29, we started to break the rules: we decided to meet face-to-face; we had lunch; we hugged. Ten days after that, I went to her apartment for the weekend. It felt like an old-school sleepover. It was great.

I'd been dating my boyfriend for only five months when COVID hit New York. He invited me to leave the city and quarantine with his parents in their summer home. I decided to go for a week. I packed up a small bag. It turned into two months. We spend all our time together, and it feels like our relationship went fast-forward—like we've been together for years. **The hardest part is that we have to have the quietest sex we can.** The bed squeaks badly. We have to invent positions where it doesn't make any noise. Mostly we start laughing, and that covers up the squeaks. We've had sex a few times outside, which was fun. I think it's a pretty good sign that we can spend 24/7 together, also with his parents, under the extremely stressful conditions of a pandemic, and still have a great time.

People in relationships are much more willing to cheat now because they're like, *Fuck it, it's the end of the world.* I had one experience with a guy—we are just friends, and we've complimented each other on being hot before. But since quarantine, we are doing it more regularly and sending pictures back and forth to each other. It's really like, *Fuck it—live your life how you want to.* I've had this happen to me with two people. One has a girlfriend who is quarantining with him, and the other is married. **But that's not stopping them from having virtual sex with me.**

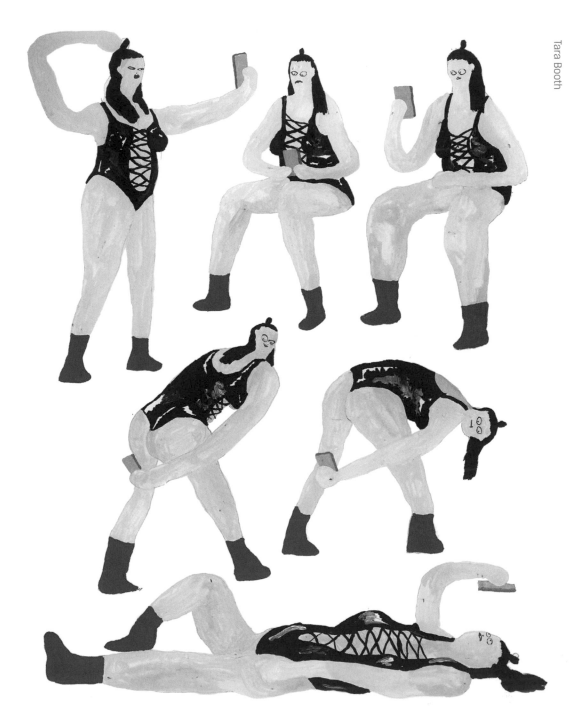

I identify as straight. I had one queer experience when I was fourteen, but that's it. In quarantine, though, I've been DMing with this woman. We are flirting, and I am beyond obsessed with her. Now I really want to sleep with a woman. Specifically, her. **I think being in quarantine is making me want to experience all the things I haven't yet.** So I'm looking forward to having a queer experience when we're out of this.

I'm at an age where they tell you you've really slid off the fertility cliff. Or you're about to. **Like every month, your reproductive insides are aging rapidly.** My partner and I were thinking we'd try for a baby and then *wham,* the 'rona hits. At first I read all of these articles that were like, *There will be a corona baby boom.* And I was like, *Okay, cool—maybe that will be us!* Then I read all of these other articles that were like, *Do not conceive a child now, you morons!* It's not like I'm thirty and can just wait thirty-six months until there's a vaccine to make a baby.

I called each family member one by one across the country. The World Health Organization had declared a pandemic only hours before. At the end of each conversation, I fumbled through the words, *Here's some good news...*

I had been pregnant twice before, both resulting in miscarriage. "Everything is good, despite it all," I said out loud to convince myself it was true. It was January in Minneapolis when I found out I was pregnant for the third time. My first trimester was dark and nauseous, during the kind of winter that seems to have no end in sight. Suddenly the light began to linger in the evenings, and my body slowly shifted to more vertical angles. The beginning of my second trimester coincided with the instant onset of worldwide panic. Just as I emerged from those early months of sickness and fatigue, the news reports rapidly escalated, ringing nonstop in my ears. A permanent blue light always shone in my eyes. All the while, my body, in automatic effort, nurtured its own thriving and untouchable miracle.

Things changed fast. First immediate unemployment with no date of return, then delayed or canceled midwife appointments with no reschedule in sight. All of this soaked heavily in a fog of confinement and a sudden fear of others. Human connection—my village, my web—had come to be my refuge,

and within hours it seemed to reveal itself as my greatest threat. *And worse,* my mind wondered constantly, *Could I unknowingly be a host to this virus?* Disinfectant wipes were rationed for doorknobs, key fobs, and steering wheels; essential whole foods and omega-filled provisions were sprayed down and scrubbed; piles of mail and delivered packages of vitamins sat untouched for days. My hands remained raw with a shriveled helpless ness that no soap or sanitizer could remove.

As the weeks turned to months, I watched my belly and breasts swell with life, a ripening that left me in awe of myself. I watched my thighs stretch and expand, watched my own chest rise and fall, filled with the force of my breath—the one power I held in my control.

There are endless tragedies that a pandemic brings about and leaves in its wake. There are also incredible moments of calm and profound hope for what remains. The paradox of nature's cruelty swirling around me while miraculous healing is taking place within me—that is not lost. It is a humble reminder that I am small, but I am mighty. And I, like so many others, can find strength in uncertainty.

I create a new mantra for myself: *Everything is good, because of it all,* I repeat in preparation for giving birth.

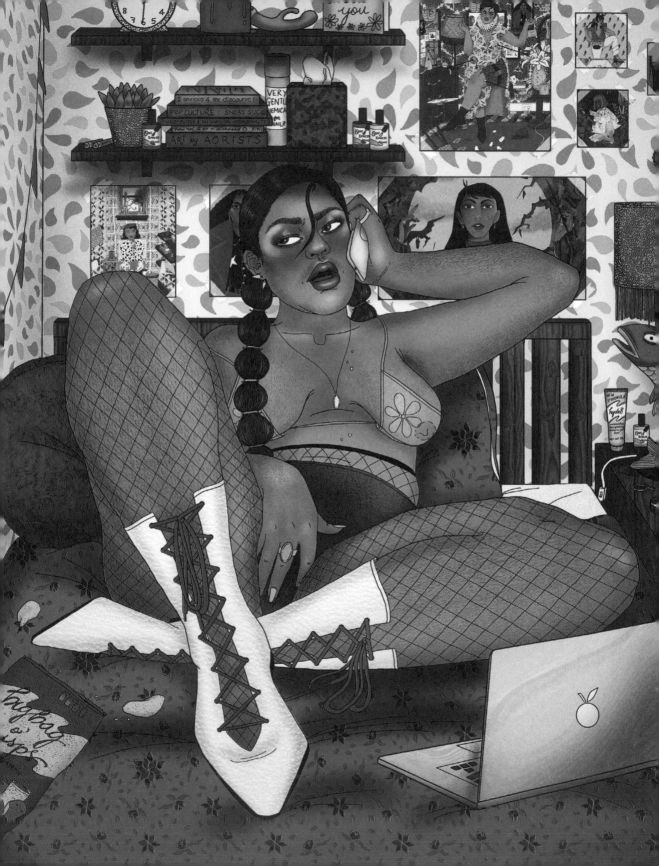

I am creating so much sex content in quarantine. I am sexting now more than ever. I think people are hornier. I'm hornier for sure, but it also feels like people are more open to being horny together. I'm sending more photos of myself to people, but I also started sending people audio of me masturbating. It's like a little podcast of me coming.

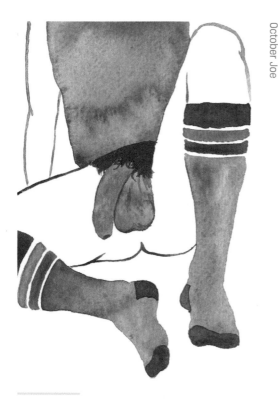

October Joe

Before COVID-19, I was a college student burned-out on my broken heart. **I live so intensely in the way that I care about people, and it felt like no one was giving me what I deserved.** I was living alone and wanted to try six months of no dating, of independence, but that was not supposed to mean no sex.

Then COVID-19 came.

At first I was quarantined alone, and I found myself loving it: taking baths and drinking wine and dancing with myself. Eventually, they closed our student housing, and I returned to live with my parents. Home is a deeply unhappy place for me, and with life and dating on pause I felt stuck. I had to remember *This is what I wanted—this is the opportunity to learn to be enough for myself and my days.*

I've found a new sense of sexuality for these times. I always thought sex had to be with a partner, but I'm finding you can experience it on your own, through your own foreplay and touch and imagination. It is an incredible discovery on my path to independence. I wanted to share.

My husband and I like to do this thing where when I get out of the shower, I slap him in the face with my boobs—which are really big. Anyway, when our kid was in school (like, when there was no pandemic happening) he would never see us do that, because usually we'd drop our kid off and go for a run, and then I'd shower, come out, and slap my husband in the face with my boobs.

I have no idea why we do this. But we do. Since we've been sheltering in place, we've done it less.

But this one time during quarantine, I came out of the shower and my husband was there in the kitchen, so I went up to him and I was like, "You've been a bad boy," and then he bent down and I slapped him back and forth with my boobs. And of course, our kid is standing right there. **He just looks at us and says, "I wish I had boobs—they look so cool."**

My best friend (and the guy I'm dating) was paroled after fifteen years at the end of March—he was paroled to a country on lockdown. We were supposed to see each other that first weekend, but NYC was already on stay-at-home orders. It's been two months now. Thinking it was going to be a short quarantine, he wanted to wait for anything sexual—no naked photos or videos, just talking and FaceTime. But about a month in, with no end in sight, things changed. We've gotten into making shower videos for each other, sexting, and audio messages. **It's fascinating to watch him adapt to the technology, considering the last phone he had before prison was a flip Razr.**

SOME SEXY NOVELS

by Emma Straub illustrations by Julia Rothman

Books can be sexy in different ways, of course, but what these books have in common, and so I suppose what I'm learning about my own feelings about sexiness, is that they all have the thrill of discovery, and of occasional wild abandoning of our thinking (and overthinking) brains. They don't all end well, but that would be a different list altogether, wouldn't it?

It all has to start somewhere.

Love Victorian novels, but wonder where all the lesbians are and want people to take off their clothes and have sex? Oh yes please.

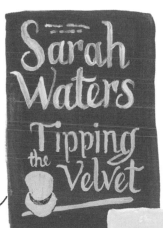

Morrison was a master of so much, including sex, and this book has some incredible moments of ecstatic abandon.

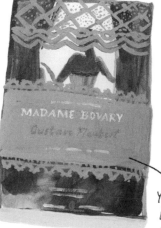

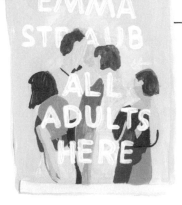

You should reread the Davis translation, if for the sex scenes alone. The carriage ride!

This is perhaps cheating, but hear me out — I've heard it said that the test for writing a good sex scene is it the author herself feels aroused, and I did.

So here I am. I won't tell you which scene, you'll have to read the whole book.

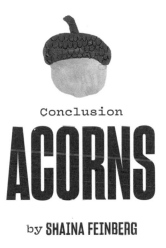

Conclusion

ACORNS

by SHAINA FEINBERG

I thought this essay would be about body dysmorphic disorder, but instead it's going to be about acorns. Sort of.

Let me explain. First of all, body dysmorphic disorder—or BDD, as I like to call it—is a condition where a person focuses on a flaw or flaws in their appearance to the point of obsession. It's something I've struggled with for a very long time. For some people, it's their hair or nose or skin that they focus on. For me it's always been more fluid. Not just one body part, but all of them. I would scrutinize my entire body in any reflective surface I could find—teakettles, butter knives, windows.

And, of course, mirrors. Mirrors were my mortal enemy.

This twisted mindset might seem like something you could easily fix, but it hasn't been. And I can't even begin to tally all of the hours, probably years, I've lost to this condition. So many things I didn't do because I wasn't physically good enough.

Instead of talking about it earnestly with people, I would joke about it. I'd tell people, "I think I look like Robert De Niro," and they'd laugh. But inside I was like, *No, really—that's what I see!* (And things could be worse— he's a very handsome man—but it's a strange thing to think as a young girl and as a woman.)

Anyway, this essay isn't going to be about BDD anymore. Because now it's about acorns.

A few months back, I was lying in bed with my kid, Monte, who had just turned four. We were reading a book called *Hector the Collector* by Emily A. Beeny, which is about a dog-boy who collects acorns. Some of the acorns are smooth, some are knobby, some green and some brown. In it is a refrain that goes, "They were all different, they were all the same, they were all beautiful." When I finished reading the book, Monte looked up at me and said, "Mama, I want a sister."

I'm not entirely sure how a book about an acorn collector created this desire in him, but it had. Maybe the idea of a collection of things made him feel lonely. After all, he was only one person—one acorn.

I decided to brush it off, and I said something to him like, "Okay, I'll see what I can do." I thought that would satisfy him, but it didn't. Instead he turned his little face to me, placed his tiny hand on my arm and asked, "How do you make a sister?"

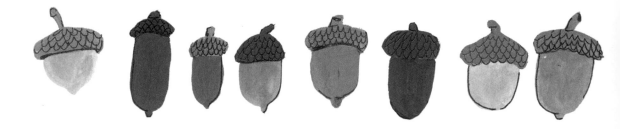

At this point I recognized I had two options: I could tell him something like, *It's complicated, and I'll tell you later.* Or I could try my best to explain how one might actually make a person.

This kind of thing isn't really in my wheelhouse. First of all, I never took sex ed because it wasn't offered in the New York City public schools I attended. And second, I'm no body expert. But I *am* a human adult, so over the years I've pieced together how a person is made. And I was fine with the fact that whatever I told Monte would be anecdotal.

So I said to him, "Well, you take some stuff from daddy and some stuff from me, and we combine it, and then some things happen inside me, and nine to ten months later a person comes out either from my vagina or my stomach."

When I'd finished my explanation, he sat up and said, "Let's do it right now! I'll go get the stuff from daddy!" He was halfway off the bed before I could stop him.

"Wait, hold on," I said. "You can't just get the stuff from daddy." (Although I guess he could, but it seemed like a lot for a Tuesday night, so I told him to hold off.)

He wasn't satisfied. "I want a sister," he whined. "A sister with a penis."

Before I started working on this book, I would have told him something totally binary and closed off. I would have said, "That's impossible." But since working on this book, I know that isn't the case. So instead I said, "Okay, maybe. It's definitely a possibility. But let's table it for now."

I don't know who's to blame for my views on sex and bodies—probably some combination of TV/movies/books/magazines/my parents? Whoever's outdated views I walked around with for most of my life are responsible for many of the shitty things I've thought and done—to myself and to others. These views of "how things should be" are responsible for the hateful things I've said to myself over the years. For most of my life, I have had a narrow-minded view of what a woman is—what she looks like, what she feels like, what parts she has, what's beautiful or ugly about her, what's acceptable. That's what I walked around with. That's what was at the root

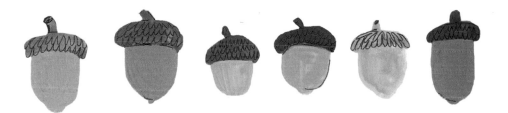

of my own struggles. But what a limited way of seeing the world! So tiny was my vision of what a woman should be, there was no space to be me.

Only once I started collaborating with Julia Rothman on this book was my limited worldview challenged and opened up. I met with so many people face-to-face, talked to them on the phone, read the stories they contributed to our website. So many different perspectives and experiences.

As I listened to and read these stories, I felt such compassion for these people. How incredible to be human! How complex! Being exposed to so many heartfelt stories made me feel more compassion for myself. I started to see my body, my life, through eyes of love. After all, I was just a human too. Just an acorn.

After months of working together on the book, I couldn't help thinking that Julia and I had become collectors. We had made a collection—not of acorns, but of stories. Stories about sex and bodies. Stories that were funny, sad, terrifying. We had collected hundreds of them. All of them were different. All of them were the same. All of them are beautiful.

ARTIST DIRECTORY

SOUFIANE ABABRI..................138, 140
@soufianeababri

ALVIN ARMSTRONG...................... 28
@eyesrevive

RACHELLE BAKER...................... 21
@indoorcatgirl

HANNAH BARCZYK.................. 74, 246
@hannabarczyk

HELEN BEARD......................46
@helenbeardart

KELLY BJORK 36
@kelly_bjork

KAYE BLEGVAD.......................... 61, 241
@kayeblegvad

TARA BOOTH...................... 201, 260
@tarabooth

JON BURGERMAN................... 100–101
@jonburgerman

HYE JIN CHUNG...................37, 181
@hyejinchung8

JOSH COCHRAN 114, 149, 158, 166
@joshcochran

LISA CONGDON 88
@lisacongdon

BRANCHE COVERDALE...............35, 151
@branchecoverdale

TIO CUCHILLOS...................58, 91, 99
@tiocuchillos

JOHN CUNEO...................30, 141, 188
@johncuneo3

EDWARD CUSHENBERRY.................162
@edwardcushenberry

ARRINGTON DE DIONYSO 87
@arringtondedionyso

CHIOMA EBINAMA......................219
@chiomaaaaaa

JON-MICHAEL FRANK 70
@jonmichaelfrank

SIOBHAN GALLAGHER...............32, 206
@siogallagher

JOHANNA GOODMAN 186
@johannagoodman

LEAH GOREN 209
@leahreenagoren

IRIS GOTTLIEB.............................89
@irisgottlieb

JASJYOT SINGH HANS 49, 175
@jasjyotjasjyot

DAVID HEATLEY...................94–95
@davidheatley

JASON ADAM KATZENSTEIN 75, 220
@j.a.k._

ANSHIKA KHULLAR 264
@aorists

KAREN KORNEGAY 238
@karenbarrettdesigns

ELENI KOUMI...................... 45, 131
@loukoumh

JENNY KROIK 256
@jkroik

LUKE KRUGER-HOWARD 19, 132
@andsoluke

HYESU LEE.............................258
@heyheysu

SLOANE LEONG.........................216
@sloaneleong

OHNI LISLE.................113, 154, 210
@ohnilisle

ADRIANA LOZANO 153
@adriana_lozano_roman

JOHN F. MALTA 123, 146
@johnfmalta

LILIAN MARTINEZ......................110
@bfgf

GEORGE McCALMAN.............167, 176
@mccalmanco

ALEX EBEN MEYER 56
@alexebenmeyer

ROMAN MURADOV............43, 116, 125
@roman_m

OCTOBER JOE 27, 159, 264
@october.joe

DANIELLE ORCHARD 31
@daniorchard

SOPHIE PAGE 18
@ladle_gull

CARISSA POTTER 72, 230
@peopleiveloved

JAIK PUPPYTEETH 179, 257
@puppyteeth

CASEY ROONAN 120
@caseyroonan

FARSHID SHAFIEY.................55, 165
@farshid_shafiey

ATIEH SOHRABI...............40, 126, 195
@atiehsohrabi

JEREMY SORESE 83, 129, 137
@jeremy_sorese

AGATHE SORLET......................... 47, 164
@agathesorlet

MANJIT THAPP..............................22
@manjitthapp

TURDLUV aka WILL VARNER..168–171
@willvarnercomics

JULIA WERTZ 222–225
@juliajwertz

LOVEIS WISE 66
@loveiswiseillu

DAVE ZACKIN 142
@davezackin

OLIMPIA ZAGNOLI 245
@olimpiazagnoli

VIRGINIA ZAMORA 161
@vee_vees

MELEK ZERTAL..........................64
@melekzertal

BALINT ZSAKO 59, 214
@balintzsako

ACKNOWLEDGMENTS

We did it!

(Thanks to the help of A LOT of people!)

We have so many people to thank...here they are in no particular order.

Thank you to all of the people who submitted stories to the website, who DM'd us, emailed us, who talked to us on street corners, in parks, on boardwalks, on the beach. Thank you for sharing—this book wouldn't exist without you. And extra thank you to... Emma Brodie, Michael Szczerban, Kate Woodrow, Jenny Volvovski, Nicky Guerreiro, Ren Khodzhayev, Chris Compeau, Wendy MacNaughton, Matt Lamothe, Eron Hare, Jessica Rothman, Jane Rothman, Jack Rothman, Mary Feinberg, Paul Feinberg, Chris Manley, Monte "Rock" Manley, Jacob Curtz, Rachel Howling Smith, Julie Showers, Shaniqwa Jarvis, Sara Nichols, Patti Smith, Jason Katzenstein, Dusty Bryndal, Drae Campbell, Rakic Evans, Jessie Strauss, Biba von Speyr, Santtu Mustonen, Marlo Thomas, Agnes Varda, Marsha P. Johnson, Gloria Steinem, Harvey Milk, Planned Parenthood, Hamilton Boardman, Phil Quinaz, Jeff Seal, Karolena Theresa, *Our Bodies, Ourselves*, Judy Blume, VC Andrews, Rob Wilson, Cheryl Dunye, Caroline Paul, Fin Lee, Jude Dry, Gretta Keene, Jon Burgerman, Trudy Beers, Rudy the Pooch, Oscar Lovinglife Shortbits, Mel Brooks, Anne Bancroft, Sarah Silverman, Madeline Kahn, Lynn Shelton, Anelle Miller, Siobhan Dooley, Lis Durkin, Seena Ghaznavi, Julia Child, Anne Frank, Ava Duvernay, Desiree Akhavan, Gina Duncan, Jerry Seinfeld, David Hockney, Robert Rauschenberg, Jason Polan, Kuye Youngblood, Rodrigo Honeywell, Alix, Jon, Jacob, Hannah and Noah Sherman, Rina Kushnir, Zackins, Michelle Hurst, Len Small, Rachael Cole, Leah Goren, Gabe Balkan, Meagan Bennett, Peter Buchanan-Smith, Lee Ann Adams, Jess Rosenkranz, Alvin Armstrong, Kuni Quimby, Harrison Allen, Elaine May, Ishtar, Tamara Jenkins, Julia Louis-Dreyfus, Nadine Thornhill, Alison Roman, New York Nico, Doss Alexander, Michelle Hope, thank you to Julia for involving me in this amazing project, thank you to Shaina for coming along on the journey. xo

ABOUT THE AUTHORS

JULIA ROTHMAN and SHAINA FEINBERG are constant collaborators. Their illustrated column, Scratch, runs every other Sunday in the *New York Times*. They have also collaborated on illustrated stories for *The New Yorker, Topic,* and other publications. JULIA is the author and/or illustrator of twelve books, including *Nature Anatomy, Ladies Drawing Night,* and *Hello, New York.* In 2017, she cofounded—with Wendy MacNaughton—Women Who Draw, an open directory of female-identifying illustrators, artists, and cartoonists. SHAINA is a writer/director who has created content for the *New York Times,* IFC, Audible, *Refinery29,* First Look Media, *This American Life,* and BRIC TV. In 2019, Shaina was named by *IndieWire* as one of twenty-five queer filmmakers to watch. Both Julia and Shaina live in Brooklyn.